Pharmaceutics-I
(General and Dispensing Pharmacy)

For B.Pharm Students

**According to Education Regulation of
Pharmacy Council of India and
All India Council for Technical Education**

Pharmaceutics-I
(General and Dispensing Pharmacy)

For B.Pharm Students

According to Education Regulation of Pharmacy Council of India and All India Council for Technical Education

Ashok K. Gupta

M.Pharm (Pharmaceutics)

Ex Head of Department, Pharmacy,
Govt. Polytechnic for Women, Chandigarh

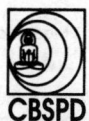

CBSPD

CBS Publishers & Distributors Pvt Ltd

New Delhi • Bengaluru • Chennai • Kochi • Kolkata • Lucknow • Mumbai
Hyderabad • Jharkhand • Nagpur • Patna • Pune • Uttarakhand

Pharmaceutics-I
General & Dispensing Pharmacy

ISBN: 978-81-239-1635-4

First Edition: 2008
Reprint: 2009, 2013, 2015, 2016, 2018, 2019, 2021, 2023, **2025**

Published by Satish Kumar Jain and Produced by Varun Jain for

CBS Publishers & Distributors Pvt Ltd
4819/XI Prahlad Street, 24 Ansari Road, Daryaganj, New Delhi 110 002, India.   4819/XI Prahlad Street, 24 Ansari Road, Daryaganj, New Delhi 110 002, India.
Ph: 23289259, 23266861   Website: www.cbspd.com
                                     e-mail: delhi@cbspd.com
Corporate Office: 204 FIE, Industrial Area, Patparganj, Delhi 110 092
Ph: 011-4934 4934   Fax: 011-4934 4935   e-mail: publishing@cbspd.com;
                                          publicity@cbspd.com

Branches

- **Bengaluru:** Seema House 2975, 17th Cross, K.R. Road, Banasankari 2nd Stage, Bengaluru 560 070, Karnataka
  Ph: +91-80-26771678/79   Fax: +91-80-26771680   e-mail: bangalore@cbspd.com
- **Chennai:** 7, Subbaraya Street, Shenoy Nagar, Chennai 600 030, Tamil Nadu, India
  Ph: +91-44-26680620/26681266   Fax: +91-44-42032115   e-mail: chennai@cbspd.com
- **Kochi:** 42/1325, 1326, Power House Road, Opp KSEB, Power House, Ernakulam 682 018, Kochi, Kerala, India
  Ph: +91-484-4059061-65, 67   Fax: +91-484-4059065   e-mail: kochi@cbspd.com
- **Kolkata:** 147, Hind Ceramics Compound, 1st Floor, Nilgunj Road, Belghoria, Kolkata-700056, West Bengal, India
  Ph: +033-25633055, 033-25633056   e-mail: kolkata@cbspd.com
- **Lucknow:** Basement, Khushnuma Complex, 7 Meerabai Marg (Behind Jawahar Bhawan), Lucknow-226001, UP, India
  Ph: +91-522-4000032   e-mail: tiwari.lucknow@cbspd.com
- **Mumbai:** PWD Shed, Gala no 25/26, Ramchandra Bhatt Marg, Next to JJ Hospital Gate no. 2, Opp. Union Bank of India Noorbaug, Mumbai-400009, Maharashtra, India
  Ph: 022-66661880/89   e-mail: mumbai@cbspd.com

Representatives

Hyderabad	0-9885175004	**Jharkhand**	0-9811541605	**Nagpur**	0-9421945513
Patna	0-9334159340	**Pune**	0-9923910676	**Uttarakhand**	0-9716462459

Printed at SRK Graphics, Shahdhara, Delhi, India

Preface

With the introduction of new syllabus by the Pharmacy Council of India and All India Council for Technical Education and various universities of respective States of the country a number of authors have come up with various books on the subject of pharmaceutics under different headings like Dispensing and General Pharmacy, Dispensing and Hospital Pharmacy, Dispensing and Community Pharmacy but none of the books meet the required material of the subject. Looking into the difficulties faced by the teachers and students of B.Pharm the author has ventured to compile the subject matter in this book which will prove useful to all concerned, respectable teachers and dear students.

I am highly thankful to all the teachers and students of whole of the country and abroad for appreciating the work done for this book and earlier books written by me.

Necessary encouragement, criticism and comments for further improvement of the book will be respectfully received and acknowledged.

My thanks are due to Sh. Satish Kumar Jain and Sh. Vinod Kumar Jain and whole team of M/s CBS Publishers & Distributors for their keen interest and painstaking efforts in bringing out the present volume of this book in a short span of time in spite of their very busy schedule.

January 2008   **Ashok K. Gupta**

v

Contents

Introduction, History and Scope of Pharmacy

EVOLUTION OF PHARMACY

Since the time of homosapiens the ailments, physical and mental, were treated with medicines. Medicines rarely occur in nature in their most useful form. First of all the drugs containing active ingredients are collected, processed and prepared for including into the formulations of medicaments. Since the dawn of humanity their system of collecting, processing and preparation is still being used.

Even today their system is being used to gain increased control over our lives to make them better and longer. Old ideas are mixed with new concepts which can lead patients into trouble.

A complete world history of how increased drug knowledge medical progress, commerce, technology and professional development came together to produce modern pharmacy and newer life-saving drugs have been evolved which have directly influenced the lives of millions of patients. Drugs such as insulin have kept thousands alive. Antibiotics and chemotherapeutic agents have saved thousands and thousands of lives. The simple fact that all medicines become useful through pharmacy and such medicines have developed a primary concern for the profession_ of pharmacy. Although pharmacy as a skill is perhaps as old as the stone age of making stone implements, this practice is recognised as about 1000 years old.

PREHISTORIC PHARMACY

Prehistoric people gathered plants for medicinal purpose. By hit and trial methods they gained knowledge of healing properties of certain natural substances which grew with the passage of time. The knowledge gained by tribals was kept a secret. Some of the medicinal which were sometimes used as food, spices or charms were apparently so widespread that it hindered any necessity for a special class of drug gatherers and keepers. The art of primitive pharmacy was mastered by all who practised the domestic medicine.

WHAT IS PHARMACY

Pharmacy is the art and science of preparing and dispensing medications and providing drug-related information to the public. It is concerned with reading of prescriptions, compounding, packing in suitable/ appropriate container, labelling and dispensing of drugs. The mission of pharmacy is to serve the suffering mankind and society.

For this purpose, a pharmacist is the right person to look all these aspects because he is educated and trained for this job. They are experts on medication. Pharmacists are considered the most suitable members of healthcare team. Moreover, he can be approached easily whenever need arises because he is the first source of assistance and can render advice on many ailments and healthcare matters.

EDUCATION

Previously diploma in pharmacy was the basic qualification for registration as a pharmacist but now the qualification for registration as a pharmacist has been raised to B.Pharmacy by Pharmacy Council of India (PCI) and All India Council for Technical Education (AICTE). Here the students of pharmacy are taught different subjects like pharmaceutics, pharmacology, industrial pharmacy, pharmacognosy, medicinal chemistry, biopharmaceutics and clinical pharmacy. Courses in social and administrative pharmacy as well as pharmacy law are also required to be studied during the course. Some other courses are becoming more prominent such as hospital pharmacy, nuclear pharmacy and management and various research specialities in the pharmaceutical industry.

SCOPE

Pharmaceutical education offers various opportunities to pharmacists with advanced degrees in any of the professional specialities. Increasing enrolments and changes in curricula at colleges to meet the employment needs of the future result in an increased need for college level trained teachers/instructors. Potentially higher salaries, more freedom for doing research and publications of the research work in educational/scientific journals, independence of action and cultural surroundings in pharmaceutical education make teaching quite attractive as compared to education in other fields. Moreover, in pharmacy line there is a great scope of advancement for all spheres.

Industrial pharmacy offers opportunities to pharmacists with degree level qualification for employment in various fields of pharmacy. The largest number of pharmacists are involved in marketing and administration. Some manufacturers employ pharmacists as their professional service representatives to educate physicians and pharmacists about the manufacturer's products. This can be a rewarding career for persons with good personality and motivation which proves for his ability and very good salary and promotion. Pharmacists with masters degree in pharmacy and business administration or additional degrees in law find better opportunities in pharmaceutical industry in marketing, sales and legal departments. With all these qualifications the pharmacist can serve in production and quality control and can be absorbed at various supervisory positions to run the affairs of the pharmaceutical industry in a proper and appropriate manner.

Since there are large opportunities in pharmacy profession that is why the people are attracted more to get a professional degree in pharmacy so as to absorb themselves at most valuable and rewarding positions. Due to all these qualities pharmacy profession is respected and gaining popularity in the field of education because by joining profession of pharmacy one can serve the suffering mankind and ailing humanity.

PHARMACOPOEIAS AND FORMULARIES

The books containing the standards for drugs and other related substances are known as pharmacopoeias and formularies; collectively these books are known as the drug compendia. The pharmacopoeias or the formularies contain a list of drugs and other related substances regarding their source, descriptions, tests, formulas for preparing the same, action and uses, doses, storage conditions, etc. These books are prepared under the authority of the governments of the respective countries. The word pharmacopoeias is derived from the Greek words pharmakon, meaning a drug, and poieo, meaning to make. Literally it means that it is a list of medicinal substances, crude drugs and formulae for making preparations from them.

These books are revised from time to time so as to introduce the latest information available as early as possible after they become established. In order to introduce new products and to keep the size of book within reasonable limits it becomes necessary to omit certain less frequently used drugs and pharmaceutical adjuvants from each new edition of the book. Therefore, in each new edition of these books certain new monographs are added while older ones are deleted.

For the preparation of these books the expert opinion of medical practitioners, teachers and pharmaceutical manufacturers is obtained.

CLASSIFICATION

The drug compendia are classified as:
1. Official compendia
2. Non-official compendia

1. Official Compendia

Official compendia are the compilations of drugs and other related substances which are recognised as legal standards of purity, quality and strength by a government agency of respective countries of their origin. Official compendia include British Pharmacopoeia, British Pharmaceutical Codex, Indian Pharmacopoeia, United States Pharmacopoeia, National Formulary, The State Pharmacopoeia of USSR and pharmacopoeias of other countries.

2. Non-official Compendia

The books other than official drug compendia which are used as secondary reference sources for drugs and other related substances are known as non-official drug compendia. These include Merck Index, Remington's Pharmaceutical Sciences, The United States Dispensatory, etc.

OFFICIAL DRUG COMPENDIAS

1. National Formulary of India

For the compilation of National Formulary of India a committee known as National Formulary Committee was constituted in November 1956 who was assigned the work to compile this formulary. The opinions of medical associations, hospitals, teaching institutions and leading manufacturers in the country were invited and finalised by the committee. It was printed in India by the Manager, Government of India Press, Simla in 1960.

2. Pharmacopoeia of India (The Indian Pharmacopoeia)

In 1946 the Government of India published the pharmacopoeial list which served as a supplement to British Pharmacopoeia. This list included the drugs which were of substantial medicinal value and were later on included in the pharmacopoeia. After the publication of this list, the Government of India constituted a permanent Indian Pharmacopoeia Committee in 1948. This committee was assigned the work to prepare Indian Pharmacopoeia and to keep it uptodate. The first edition of Indian Pharmacopoeia was published in 1955 and a supplement of it was published in 1960.

The work of revision of the Indian Pharmacopoeia as well as the compilation of new edition was taken up simultaneously under the chairmanship of Dr. B.N. Ghosh, Professor of Pharmacology, R.G. Kar Medical College, Calcutta, who died in 1958. After Dr. B.N. Ghosh, Dr. B. Mukerji, Director, Central Drug Research Institute, Lucknow, was appointed as chairman of the Indian Pharmacopoeia Committee. The second edition of the Indian Pharmacopoeia was published in 1966 and a supplement of it was published in 1975.

On 30th June 1978, the Indian Pharmacopoeia Committee was reconstituted by the Government of India, Ministry of Health and Family Welfare, under the chairmanship of Dr. Nitya Nand, Director, Central Drug Research Institute, Lucknow. This committee was assigned the work for the preparation of the third edition of the Indian Pharmacopoeia. A working group was constituted by the committee to prepare monographs, appendices and general notes which were finalised by the Pharmacopoeia Committee. The same were published in the form of the Pharmacopoeia of India in 1985, in two volumes, volume I and volume II by the Controller of Publications, Delhi on behalf of

Government of India, Ministry of Health and Family Welfare. The volume I contains legal notices, preface, acknowledgements, introduction, general notices and monographs from A to P. The volume II contains monographs from Q to Z, appendices, contents of appendices and index.

For the preparation of Pharmacopoeia of India, the pharmacopoeias of other countries like British, Europe, United States, USSR, Japan, the National Formulary (U.S.A.) and Merck Index were consulted. The persons working in pharmaceutical industry, drug control laboratories, research and teaching institutions also actively participated.

Under the Drugs and Cosmetics Act 1940, the Indian Pharmacopoeia is an official book which contains the standards for drugs and other related substances included in the pharmacopoeia. The drugs and other related substances prepared by pharmaceutical manufacturers must comply with these standards.

3. British Pharmacopoeia

The responsibility of publishing the British Pharmacopoeia has rested upon the General Medical Council since the Medical Act 1858. The provisions and duties of this council are contained in section 47 of the Medical Act, 1956. According to the recommendations of the Macmillan Committee, the work of preparing new editions of the pharmacopoeia was entrusted by the General Medical Council to the Pharmacopoeia Commission.

The Pharmacopoeia Commission is reconstituted from time to time for a period which corresponds to the period during which a new edition of the British Pharmacopoeia is prepared and published. Since 1948 the new edition of the British Pharmacopoeia is published at intervals of five years i.e. 1948, 1953, 1958, 1963, 1968, 1973. After 1973 the new edition was published in 1980 and then in 1988. In addition to the publication of the pharmacopoeia, the addendums are also published from time to time in between two main editions.

The British Pharmacopoeia 1980, thirteenth edition and 1988, the fourteenth edition was published by Her Majesty's Stationery Office for the Health Ministers on the recommendations of the Medicines Commission in accordance with the Medicines Act 1968.

British Pharmacopoeia is the source of official standards for drugs in the United Kingdom and other parts of the world. Generations of pharmaceutical students were brought up to regard the pharmacopoeia as the main source of all their pharmaceutical knowledge. Nowadays the pharmacopoeia also provides knowledge about pharmaceutical products regarding standards and methods of analysis to be employed.

4. British Pharmaceutical Codex

It was in 1903 that the Council of the Pharmaceutical Society of Great Britain decided to prepare a reference book for the use of medical practitioners and dispensing pharmacists. The first edition of the British Pharmaceutical Codex was published in 1907. The subsequent revisions of this codex were published in 1911, 1923, 1934, 1949, 1954, 1959, 1963, 1968, 1973.

On the request of British Pharmacopoeia Commission, the Council of the Pharmaceutical Society agreed in 1959 for the publication of Codex to coincide with that of the British Pharmacopoeia, so that these two books i.e. British Pharmaceutical Codex and British Pharmacopoeia should come into effect on the same dates.

The British Pharmaceutical Codex differs from British Pharmacopoeia in that:

(a) It contains many more drugs and preparations; some may be included in advance of the pharmacopoeia and may acquire the official status while other drugs may have been included in the former editions of pharmacopoeia but now they are retained in the Codex because they are still commonly used.

(b) It provides standards for drugs, surgical dressings and pharmaceutical preparations not included in the British Pharmacopoeia.

(c) It provides information on the actions and uses of drugs, their undesirable effects, precautions and the treatment of poisoning.

(d) It contains formulae, method of preparation, dose, container and storage conditions of most of the preparations which are still extemporaneously prepared in the pharmacy and dispensed by the pharmacists. These preparations include mixtures, powders, eye drops, ear drops, liniments, lotions, ointments, creams, pastes, suppositories, etc.

5. The United States Pharmacopoeia

The United States Pharmacopoeia and the National Formulary (USP-NF) are recognised as official compendia and are used as reference books for determining the strength, quality, purity, packaging and labelling of drugs and other related articles.

The United States Pharmacopoeia was originally published in 1820 under the authority of the United States Pharmacopoeial Convention and the National Formulary was published in 1888 under the guidance of the American Pharmaceutical Association. In 1974 the National Formulary was purchased by the United States Pharmacopoeial Convention and from 1980 onwards only one official book of drug standards was published under the heading, The United States Pharmacopoeia and The National Formulary (USP-NF).

6. Extra Pharmacopoeia (Martindale)

The Extra Pharmacopoeia was first produced in 1883 by William Martindale and is still known as "Martindale". This is an authorised reference book on drugs and is used throughout the world. It provides all sorts of latest information on drugs and medicines. The Extra Pharmacopoeia is prepared by consulting the pharmacopoeias of other countries. The twenty-eighth edition was published in December 1982. The twenty-ninth edition was published in January 1989 by direction of the Council of the Royal Pharmaceutical Society of Great Britain and prepared in the Society's Department of Pharmaceutical Sciences.

7. The Merck Index

It is an encyclopedia of chemicals, drugs and biologicals. The first edition was published in 1889 and the eleventh edition in 1989 by Merck & Co., Inc., Rahway, N.J., U.S.A.

8. The International Pharmacopoeia

The International Pharmacopoeia is published by the World Health Organisation and is particularly used in developing countries.

9. State Pharmacopoeia of the USSR

The first edition of the State Pharmacopoeia of the Union of Soviet Socialist Republics was published in 1866 in Russian language. It was followed by next editions in 1871, 1880, 1891, 1902, 1910, 1925, 1946, 1961, so on. The 9th edition was published in 1961 under the auspices of Pharmacopoeia Committee of the Ministry of Health of the USSR. Research institutes, pharmaceutical teaching institutions, industrial houses and specialists of highest qualifications were actively associated with the publication of the pharmacopoeias.

OTHER USEFUL BOOKS AND PERIODICALS

Textbooks

1. *Bentley's Textbook of Pharmaceutics*, H. Davis.
2. *Remington's Pharmaceutical Sciences*, Mack Publishing Company, Pennsylvania.
3. *Introduction to Pharmaceutical Dosage Forms*, H.C. Ansel, Lea and Febiger.
4. *Dispensing of Medication*, E.W. Martin, Mack Publishing Co.
5. *Dispensing for Pharmaceutical Students*, Cooper and Gunn, Pitman Publishing Company, London.
6. *The Theory and Practice of Industrial Pharmacy*, Leon Lachman, Varghese Publishing House, Hind Rajasthan Building, Dadar, Bombay - 400014.

Journals

1. **Indian Journal of Pharmaceutical Sciences:** It is a scientific publication of the Indian Pharmaceutical Association. It was formerly known as the Indian Journal of Pharmacy.
2. **Indian Journal of Pharmaceutical Education:** This journal is the official publication of Association of Pharmaceutical Teachers of India and is published quarterly in March, June, September and December every year.
3. **The Eastern Pharmacist:** It is published on the 15th day of every month from New Delhi located at 507, Ashok Bhawan, 93 Nehru Place, New Delhi - 110016 and published on behalf of the Eastern Pharmacist from E-38, Hauz Khas, New Delhi - 110016.
4. **American Journal of Pharmaceutical Education:** It is the official publication of American Association of Colleges of Pharmacy. Its purpose is to document pharmaceutical education and to advance it.
5. **Journal of Medicinal Chemistry:** It is published biweekly by the American Chemical Society at 1155, 16th St. N.W., Washington DC 20036.
6. **Pharma Today:** It is a monthly pharmaceutical trade magazine edited and published by G.S. Rao on behalf of Sharavathi Management Services, C5/19-24, Sector 3, P.O. Konkan Bhawan, C.B.D., New Bombay - 400614.

Prescription

Prescription is an order written by a physician, dentist or any other registered medical practitioner to a pharmacist to compound and dispense a specific medication for the patient. The order is accompanied by directions for the pharmacist that what type of preparation is to be prepared and how much is to be prepared. It is also accompanied with the directions for the patient that how much medicament is to be taken, how many times it is to be taken or at what time and how it is to be taken.

The prescription provides a common link of mutual interest between the physician, the pharmacist and the patient. It is the duty of the pharmacist to serve the medication needs of the patient according to the intention of the prescriber. It is not sufficient that the pharmacist should only compound the specific medication but he should make the patient understand about the proper administration of the drug and ensure that the patient sticks to these instructions. At the same time the pharmacist must maintain and respect the confidentiality of both the physician regarding the treatment given as well as that of the patient regarding the nature of his illness and the medication taken by him.

The prescriptions are generally written in the language of the area in which they originate but Latin words are frequently used in the prescription writing because in the olden days the medicines were written in Latin language which was understood all over the world. Still the use of Latin abbreviations in the prescription writing is very common, specially in dosage instructions.

PARTS OF A PRESCRIPTION

A complete prescription should have the following parts:

1. Date
2. Name, age, sex and address of the patient
3. Superscription
4. Inscription
5. Subscription
6. Signatura
7. Signature, address and registration number of prescriber.

1. Date

Date must be written on the prescription by the prescriber at the same time when it is written. The date on the prescription helps a pharmacist to find out the cases where prescription is brought for dispensing long time after its issue. Prescriptions containing narcotic or other habit-forming drugs must bear the date. The prescriptions should be filled within a reasonable time after it is written. If the prescription is brought for filling after two or three days from the date when it was written then the pharmacist must question if the intention of the prescriber and the needs of the patient can still be met.

2. Name, Age, Sex, and Address of the Patient

Name, age, sex, and address of the patient must be written on the prescription. If it is not written then the pharmacist himself should ask the patient about these particulars and put down at the top of the prescription. This avoids the possibility of giving the finished product to a person other than the one it is meant for. Patient's full name must be written instead of surname or the family name.

Age and sex of the patient specially in the case of children helps the pharmacist in checking the medication and the dose. Therefore there will be less danger of its being administered to the wrong member of the family or the hospital ward having similar names. The address of

---

An Example of A Typical Prescription

General Hospital

Date   14.10.2007
Name   Sh. Raman Kumar
Age   40 years
Sex   Male
Address   817, Sector-20 Chandigarh

R_x (Superscription)

Potassium Bromide   8 gm ⎫
Tincture Nux Vomica   8 ml   ⎬ (Inscription)
Chloroform Water q.s.   120 ml ⎭

Fiat mistura (Subscription)

Sig. Cochleare magnum ter in die post cibos sumenda. (Signatura)

(Signature of the Prescriber)
S.C. Aggarwal M.D.
Regd. No. 10234

---

the patient is recorded to help for any reference at a later stage, to contact the patient or to deliver the medication personally.

3. Superscription

The superscription is represented by a symbol R_x which is always written at the beginning of the prescription. In the days of mythology and superstition the symbol was considered as a prayer to Jupiter, the God of healing, for quick recovery of the patient but now this symbol is understood as an abbreviation of the Latin word recipe, meaning "take thou" or "you take".

4. Inscription

This is the main part of the prescription. It contains the names and quantities of the prescribed ingredients. The names of the ingredients are written each on a separate line, followed by the quantity ordered and the last item written is generally the vehicle or diluent. In complex prescriptions containing several ingredients the inscription is divided into three parts (a) the base or the active medicament which is intended to produce the therapeutic effect; (b) the adjuvant which is included either to enhance the action of the medicament or to make the product more palatable; (c) the vehicle which is either used to dissolve the solid substances and/or to increase the volume of the preparation for ease of administration.

Now a days only a few prescriptions are compounded by pharmacists. A majority of prescriptions are written for medications already prepared into dosage forms by industrial manufacturers. The pharmacists are only required to dispense the ready-made dosage form of drugs which has eliminated the compounding of prescriptions.

5. Subscription

This part of the prescription contains prescriber's directions to the pharmacist regarding the dosage form to be prepared and number of doses to be dispensed. Since now-a-days only a few prescriptions are compounded therefore such directions are less frequent.

6. Signatura

It is usually abbreviated as "Sig" on the prescriptions and consists of the directions to be given to the patient regarding the administration of the drug. It usually indicates the quantity of medicament or number or dosage units to be taken, how many times in a day or at what time it should be taken and the manner in which it is to be administered or applied. These instructions must be transferred to the label of the container in which the medicament is to be dispensed and ensure that the patient follows these instructions carefully.

7. Signature, Address and Registration Number of the Prescriber

All other parts of the prescription may be printed or type-written but the prescriber's name must be hand-written and should be signed with ink. This eliminates the danger of dispensing medicament on a spurious order and it authenticates the prescription. The prescriptions containing narcotic or other habit-forming drugs must bear the address and registration number of the prescriber. This identifies the special licence which a prescriber must have to prescribe the narcotic and other habit-forming drugs.

HANDLING OF PRESCRIPTION

1. Receiving
2. Reading and checking
3. Collecting the materials
4. Weighing
5. Compounding
6. Finishing.

1. Receiving

The prescription should be received from the patient by the pharmacist himself. Under no circumstances an unauthorised person should try to receive or read the prescription.

2. Reading and Checking

A brief examination of each prescription should be made immediately upon receiving it from the patient. This will tell the pharmacist about the nature of the dosage form to be prepared and he can estimate the time required for preparing it. If a long time is needed for compounding the prescription then he must tell the patient about the time required for filling the prescription so that he may wait or return after some time. In some cases the patient's name, age and address may not be written on the prescription, in such cases these informations should be enquired from the patient and put down on the prescription.

Careful examination of the prescription should be made only behind the counter, so that if there is any doubt regarding the prescription ingredients or directions or there is any error in writing the prescription, the patient should not come to know about it. If there is any doubt the pharmacist should consult the other pharmacists or the prescriber.

Every prescription should be read and understood completely before compounding it. Every word and abbreviation must be interpreted correctly. He should never guess about the meaning of an illegible or confusing word. It may lead to serious consequences. If there is any doubt he should consult the fellow pharmacists or the prescriber.

As the number of drugs available in the market are increasing, the mistakes, due to the similarity or pronunciation and spellings are also increasing. In such cases a pharmacist has to take a great care specially when the prescriptions are received orally. Examples of such drugs which look alike or sound alike are given below:

Apresoline	Priscoline
Compocillin	Ampicillin
Daricon	Darvon
Digoxin	Digitoxin
Indocin	Lincocin
Prednisone	Prednisolone
Qinine	Quinidine

Before the start of compounding the prescription, the pharmacist must ensure that what he is going to do and what type of finished product he will obtain.

3. Collecting and Weighing the Materials

Materials to be used in compounding the prescription should be collected on the left hand side of the balance and arranged in the order in which they are to be mixed. The materials which are weighed should be shifted to right hand side of the balance. This gives a mechanical check of ingredients which has been weighed. The label on every stock bottle should be read at least three times:

(a) When taken from the shelf or drawer.

(b) When the contents are removed for weighing or measuring.

(c) When the containers are returned back to its proper place.

4. Compounding

This is the most important phase in handling the prescription. In this case proper drug is dispensed in a suitable form. This can be achieved only if accuracy, cleanliness and proper techniques are observed in the preparation of any medication. Only one prescription should be compounded at one time. If two or more prescriptions are dispensed at the same time, one is likely to make serious mistakes by dispensing wrong drugs. Attention should not be diverted by talking to friends, attending the telephone or engaging in other directions.

Now a days majority of the prescriptions are written for the pre-compounded dosage forms supplied by the pharmaceutical manufacturers which require no compounding or mixing by the pharmacist. When a prescription requiring compounding is received the pharmacist should decide the calculations, special adjuvants and order of mixing then he should proceed further as described above.

5. Finishing

The compounded medicaments should be filled in suitable containers depending on the quantity of the medication to be dispensed and the method of its use. Various types of containers used in pharmacy are: round vials used for filling the unit dosage forms such as tablets and capsules; oval prescription bottles used for filling liquids of low viscosity; wide mouth bottles used for filling the liquids of high viscosity, large quantities of tablets or capsules and bulk powders; ointment jars and collapsible tubes used for filling the ointments, creams or semisolid dosage forms; dropper bottles used for dispensing the eye drops, ear drops or other liquids to be administered by drops; sifter top containers used for dispensing the powders meant to be applied externally by sprinkling etc. The container should be selected approximately of the same volume as that of the medication to be dispensed.

Most of the containers are available in various sizes, shapes, colours and compositions. They may be made up of glass, plastic or suitable metal. Most of the glass containers are made from colourless or amber coloured glass. The latter being used for dispensing light sensitive medications. Plastic containers and collapsible tubes are also widely used for dispensing various types of dosage forms.

The filled containers are suitably labelled. A good quality of paper and adhesive should be used for labelling the containers. The size of the label should be proportional to the size of the container and should be neatly hand-written or preferably typed. The following information should be written on all labels:

1. Name of the prescription
2. Name of the patient, age and sex
3. Registration number
4. Date of dispensing
5. Directions for its use
6. Expiry date, if any
7. Storage conditions
8. Name and address of the pharmacy.

The label should be placed almost in the centre leaving equal space from the bottom and top of the bottle. On collapsible tubes it should be placed near the top to avoid concealment and wrinkling as the tube is rolled up from the bottom during its use. Special adhesives should be used for fixing the labels on the collapsible tubes.

Some containers like ophthalmic ointment tubes, eye drop and ear drop bottles and other small containers which lack sufficient surface area for attaching the label may be labelled with the serial number and packed in bigger container which is properly labelled. Special directions like "For external use only." and "Shake the bottle before use." must be attached to the bottle as secondary label.

After preparing and labelling, the compounded prescription should be thoroughly examined to ensure accuracy, quality and safety of the prescription. The checker should first check the written prescription and then the contents of the container for colour, odour or any other indication for the correctness and quality of the medication. If the checker finds that the compounded prescription is correct then he must put his signatures on the prescription. Before the prescription is handed over to the patient the container must be thoroughly polished so as to remove the finger prints.

PRICING THE PRESCRIPTION

The prices of prescriptions and drugs have increased to a great extent in recent years not only due to a general rise in the prices of all goods but due to advent of newer, more powerful drugs which have been discovered and marketed only after lot of research and huge investment in the form of dollars and rupees. The cost of research must be recovered and reinvested in further research for the ultimate benefit of the public.

The charges applied to a prescription should include the costs of the ingredients including the containers and label the time of the pharmacist and other persons should also be included in the cost of prescription. The other operational costs of the department as well as reasonable margin of profit on the investments should also be included.

Once the price for a prescription has been determined the same may be recorded for future use. It will save time and energy of all the concerned persons.

LATIN TERMS AND ABBREVIATIONS
COMMONLY USED IN PRESCRIPTION WRITING

Latin term or phrase	Abbreviation	English meaning
Ad	ad.	to, up to
Ad libitum	ad. lib.	at pleasure, as desired
Admove	admov.	apply
Agita	agit.	shake, stir
Alter	alt.	the other, alternate
Alternis horis	alt. hrs.	alternate hours
Ana	a a.	of each
Ante	a.	before
Ante cibos	a.c.	before meals
Applicandus	applicand	to be applied
Aqua	aq.	water
Aqua bulliens	aq. bull.	boiling water
Aqua destillata	aq. dest.	distilled water
Auris dextra	a.d.	right ear
Auris laeva	a.l.	left ear
Auristillae	auristill	ear drops
Bis in die	b.i.d.	twice a day
Capsula	caps.	capsule
Capiat	cap.	let him take
Capiendus	capiend.	to be taken
Cataplasma	cataplasm	poultice
Charta	chart.	powder, powder paper
Cibos	cibos.	food, meals
Cochleare ⎰amplum ⎱magnum ⎰maximum	coch ⎰amp. ⎱mag. ⎰max.	one tablespoonful
Cochleare ⎰medium ⎱modicum	coch ⎰med. ⎱mod.	one desertspoonful
Cochleare ⎰minimum ⎱parvum	coch ⎰min. ⎱parv.	one teaspoonful
Collunarium	collunar.	a nose wash

(Contd.)

Latin term or phrase	Abbreviation	English meaning
Collutorium	collut.	a mouth wash
Collyrium	collyr.	an eye wash
Congius	cong; c	a gallon
Cum	c	with
Cum duplo	c. dup.	with twice as much
Cum parte aequale	c. pt. aeq.	with an equal quantity
Cyathus	cyath.	a glass
Dentur	dent.	give, let it be given
Dexter	dext.	right
Diebus alternis	dieb. alt.	every other day
Divide	div.	divide
Dolore urgente	dol. urg.	when the pain is severe
Emulsio	emul.	an emulsion
E	—	with
E. lacte	e. lact.	with milk
Ex. aqua	ex. aq.	with water
Ex. modo prescripto	e.m.p.	in the manner prescribed
Fiat, fit, fiant.	ft.	make, let it be made
Granum, grana	gr.	a grain
Gutta, guttae	gtt.	a drop, drops
Hac nocte	hac noct.	to night
Hora	h.	an hour
Hora somni	h.s.	at bed time
In dies	In. d.	daily
Inter cibos	i.c.	during meals
Injectio	Inj.	an injection
Laevo	l.	left
Levis	lev.	light
Linimentum	lin.	a liniment
Liquor	liq.	solution
Mane	m.	morning
Minimum	min.	a minim
Misce	m.	mix, let (it) be mixed
Mistura	mist.	a mixture

(Contd.)

Latin term or phrase	Abbreviation	English meaning
Mitte	mitt.	send
Mitte tales	mitt tal.	send such
Modo dicto	m. dict.	as directed, as stated
Modo prescripto	m. pres.	as prescribed
More dicto	m. dict.	in the manner prescribed
Nebula	nebul.	a spray
Nocte maneque	noct. maneq.	night and morning
Non repetatur	non rep, n.r.	do not repeat
Octarius	o.	a pint
Oculo utro	o.u.	each eye
Oculus dexter	o.d.	right eye
Oculus laevus	o.l.	left eye
Oculus sinister	o.s.	left eye
Omni	omn.	every
Omni hora	omn. hor, o.h.	every hour
Omni quadranta hora	omn. quadr. hor	every quarter of an hour
Omni quarta hora	omn. 4 hrs.	every four hours
Omni secunda hora	omn. 2 hrs.	every two hours
Omni mane	o.m.	every morning
Omni nocte	o.n.	every night
Os, oris	o.s.	mouth
Parti affecti applicandus	p.a.a.	to be applied to the affected part
Per os	p.o.	orally by mouth
Phiala prius agitata	p.p.a.	the bottle, being first shaken (i.e., attach a "Shake the bottle." label)
Post cibos	p.c.	after meals
Pro oculo laevo	p.o.l.	for the left eye
Pro dosi	—	as a dose
Pro re nata	p.r.n.	when necessary, occasionally
Pulvis	pulv	powder

(Contd.)

Latin term or phrase	Abbreviation	English meaning
Quantum sufficiat	q.s.	as much as sufficient
Quaque quarta hora	q.q.h.	every fourth hour
Quarter in die	q.i.d.	four times a day
Quotidie	quot.	Daily
Recipe	Rx	take
Secundum artum	s.a.	according to the art
Semis, Semi	ss.	half
Signa, signetur	sig.	write
Si opus sit	s.o.s.	when necessary
Solve	—	dissolve
Solutio	sol.	a solution
Statim	stat.	immediately
Sumendus	sum.	to be taken
Suppositorium	supp.	a suppository
Tabella, tabletta	tab.	a tablet
Talis, tales	tal.	such
Ter in die	t.i.d.	three times a day
Ter quotidie	—	three times daily
Tussi urgente	tuss. urg.	when the cough is troublesome
Uncia	—	an ounce
Unguentum	ung.	an ointment
Utendus	u. or utend.	to be used
Unus	i	one
Duo	ii	two
Tres	iii	three
Quatuor	iv	four
Quinque	v	five
Sex	vi	six
Septem	vii	seven
Octo	viii	eight
Novem	ix	nine
Decem	x	ten
Undecim	xi	eleven
Duodecim	xii	twelve
Quindecim	xv	fifteen

Meteorology and Calculations

CALCULATIONS INVOLVED IN DISPENSING

Before discussing the calculations which are involved in dispensing of drugs it is very necessary to have a thorough knowledge regarding weights and measures which are used in calculations. These weights and measures are discussed as follows:

Weight

It is a measure of the gravitational force acting on a body and is directly proportional to its mass. The mass remains constant and never varies because it is based on inertia whereas weight varies slightly with change in latitude, altitude, temperature and pressure. The effect of these factors is not considered unless very accurate weighings are to be done.

Measure

It is the measurement of volume of any substance. Temperature and pressure exert their effect specially on liquids and gases. The effect of these factors is only taken into consideration when accurate preparations are to be made.

There are two systems of weights and measures (a) the imperial system (b) the metric system, with which the pharmacist must be familiar.

The imperial system is an old system based on arbitrary and unrelated units, e.g., grains, drachms, ounces and gallons whereas the metric system or decimal system is based on related and rationally derived units, e.g., milligrams, grams, centimeters, meters, millilitres, litres, etc. Because of its easier calculations, greater accuracy and flexibility and use in other sciences, now a days this is the most widely used system by official agencies.

ADOPTION OF METRIC SYSTEM

In 1948 a committee on weights and measures legislation was appointed by the president of the Board of Trade to review the existing weights and measures legislation and to make recommendations thereof. In 1951 the committee published a report in which it was recommended that the apothecary system (Imperial system) should be abolished and the metric system should be adopted in its place. Therefore steps were taken to abolish the use of imperial system for all dealings in drugs and medicines and its use was declared illegal in pharmacy profession. Since 31st March 1969 pharmacists were required to carry out all dispensing work in metric system. Similarly since 3rd March 1969 it was illegal in Great Britain to use for dispensing any system of weights and measures other than the metric system.

Accordingly the first change over to the metric system appeared in the British Pharmacopoeia and British Pharmaceutical Codex published in 1963. The doses of tablets, capsules and injections were given only in metric quantities. Weights and Measures Regulations 1964 described certain equivalents in metric units that whenever strength is prescribed in the imperial units that must be dispensed according to equivalent strength in metric units.

Though the pharmacists are required to use the metric system for dispensing the prescriptions but still a large number of physicians trained to use the imperial system prescribe the drugs in the old system and some hospitals still retain it as the local standard. Some drugs are prescribed in fractional doses (1/200, 1/150, 1/100 gr). The bottles for liquids are still manufactured to contain ounce measurements rather than milliliters.

Due to the above mentioned reasons, it is still necessary to be familiar with both the systems which are described in detail as follows:

(a) Imperial System

Imperial system is divided into two systems:

1. Avoirdupois system
2. Apothecaries system.

Avoirdupois system

According to this system the standard unit for weighing is pound and all other measures of mass are derived from pound. It is represented by lb.

1 lb	= 16 oz (Avoir)	
1 lb	= 7000 grains	
1 oz	= 7000/16	= 437.5 grains

Apothecaries system

It is known as troy system. The standard weight in this system is grain.

20 grain	= 1 scruple
60 grain	= 1 drachm
480 grain	= 1 ounce (Apothe)
8 drachm	= 1 ounce (Apothe)
12 ounces (Apothe)	= 1 pound (Apothe)
5760 grain	= 1 pound (Apothe)

Abbreviations commonly used in weighing

Latin name	Symbol	English name	Equal to
Granum	gr	grain	1 grain
Scrupulus	Э	scruple	20 grains
Drachma	ʒ	drachm	60 grains
Uncia	oz	ounce (Avoir)	437.5 grains
Uncia	℥	ounce (Apothe)	480 grains
Libra	lb	pound (Avoir)	7000 grains
Libra	lb	pound (Apothe)	5760 grains

Measures of Capacity

Standard units for capacity are same in avoirdupois as well as apothecaries system. The standard unit is gallon and all other measures of capacity are derived from gallon.

1 gallon	= 160 fluid ounces	
1/4th of a gallon	= 1 quart	= 40 fl. ounce

1/8th of gallon	= 1 pint	= 20 fl. ounce
1/160th of a gallon	= 1 fl. ounce	
1/8th of one fl. ounce	= 1 fl. drachm	
1/60th of one fl. drachm	= 1 minim	
1 fluid ounce	= 480 minim	
1 fluid drachm	= 480/8	= 60 minim

Abbreviations commonly used in measures of capacity

Latin name	Symbol	English name	Equal to
Minimum	m	minim	1 minim
Fluidrachma	ʒ	fl. drachm	60 minim
Fluidunicia	ʒ	fl. ounce	480 minim
Octarius	O	pint	20 fl. ounces
Congius	C	gallon	160 fl. ounces

Metric System

Standard unit of measures of mass (weight) is kilogram and all other measures of mass are derived from kilogram.

1 Kilogram (kg)	= 1000 gm	
1 Hectogram (hg)	= 100 gm	
1 Decagram (dag)	= 10 gm	
1 Gram (gm)	= 1 gm	
1 Decigram (dg)	= 0.1 gm	= 100 mg
1 Centigram (cg)	= 0.01 gm	= 10 mg
1 Milligram (mg)	= 0.001 gm	= 1 mg
1 Microgram (mg, mcg)	= 1/1000 mg	

Measures of Capacity

Standard unit for measures of capacity (volume) is litre and all other measures of capacity are derived from litre.

1 litre (lt) = 1000 millilitre (ml)

Domestic Measures

1 drop	= 1 minim	= 0.06 ml
1 tea spoonful	= 1 fl. drachm	= 4 ml
1 desert spoonful	= 2 fl. drachm	= 8 ml
1 table spoonful	= 4 fl. drachm	= 15 ml
2 table spoonful	= 1 fl. ounce	= 30 ml

1 wine glassful	= 2 fl. ounce	= 60 ml
1 tea cupful	= 4 fl. ounce	= 120 ml
1 tumblerful	= 8 fl. ounce	= 240 ml

Conversion Factors

1 grain	= 64.8 mg	= 65 mg	(for all practical purposes)
1 drop	= 1 minim	= 0.06 ml	(for all practical purposes)
1 fl. ounce	= 29.57 ml	= 30 ml	(for all practical purposes)
1 gram	= 15.43 gr	= 15 gr	(for all practical purposes)
1 milligram	= 1/65 gr	= 1/65 gr	(for all practical purposes)
1 millilitre	= 16.23 minim	= 15 m	(for all practical purposes)
1 litre	= 33.8 fl. ounce		
1 kilogram	= 2.2 pound		

CALCULATIONS

Calculations based on density

Density in defined as the mass of a substance per unit volume. It has the units of mass over volume.

Specific gravity is the ratio of the weight of a substance in air to that of an equal volume of water. It does not have any units.

In the metric system both density and specific gravity are numerically equal. The density, weight and volume of any substance can be calculated from the following equations:

$$\text{Density} = \frac{\text{Weight}}{\text{Volume}}$$

$$\text{Weight} = \text{Density} \times \text{Volume}$$

$$\text{Volume} = \frac{\text{Weight}}{\text{Density}}$$

If any two variables are given, the third one can be calculated.

1. Calculate the weight of 120 ml of an oil whose density is 0.9624 gm/ml.

$$\text{Weight} = \text{Density} \times \text{Volume}$$
$$= 0.9624 \text{ gm/ml} \times 120 \text{ ml} = 115.488 \text{ gm}$$

2. Calculate the volume of 200 gm of glycerin. The density of glycerin is 1.25 gm/ml.

$$Volume = \frac{Weight}{Density}$$

$$= \frac{200 \text{ gm}}{1.25 \text{ gm/ml}} = 160 \text{ ml}$$

3. Calculate the weight of 1 litre of alcohol whose density is 0.816 gm/ml.

Weight = Density × Volume

$$= 0.816 \text{ gm/ml} \times 1000 \text{ ml} = 816 \text{ gm}$$

Conversions from Imperial to Metric and Metric to Imperial Systems

1. How many mg are in one grain.

Since   15.43 gr = 1 gm

$$1 \text{ gr} = \frac{1}{15.43} \text{ gm} = 0.0648 \text{ gm} = 64.8 \text{ mg}$$

∴   1 gr = 64.8 mg

2. How many grams are in 1 ounce (Apothe).

    1 ounce (Apothe) = 480 gr

Since   15.43 gr = 1 gm

$$1 \text{ gr} = \frac{1}{15.43}$$

$$480 \text{ gr} = \frac{1}{15.43} \times 480 = 31.11 \text{ gm}$$

∴   1 ounce (Apothe) = 31.11 gm

3. How many grams are in 1 ounce (Avoir).

    1 ounce (Avoir) = 437.5 gr

Since   15.43 gr = 1 gm

$$1 \text{ gr} = \frac{1}{15.43} \text{ gm}$$

$$437.5 \text{ gr} = \frac{1}{15.43} \times 437.5 = 28.35 \text{ gm}$$

∴   1 ounce (Avoir) = 28.35 gr

4. How many ml are in 1 fl. oz.

   1 fl. oz = 480 m

   16.23 m = 1 ml

   $$1 \text{ m} = \frac{1}{16.23} \text{ ml}$$

   $$480 \text{ m} = \frac{1}{16.23} \times 480 = 29.57 \text{ ml}$$

∴   1 fl. oz = 29.57 ml.

5. Convert 3 drachm into mgs.

   1 drachm = 60 gr

   3 drachm = 60 × 3 = 180 gr

   1 gr = 64.8 mg

   180 gr = 64.8 × 180 = 11664 mg

   3 drachm = 11664 mg.

6. Convert 550 mg into grains.

   64.8 mg = 1 gr

   $$1 \text{ mg} = \frac{1}{64.8} \text{ gr}$$

   $$550 \text{ mg} = \frac{1}{64.8} \times 550 = 8.48 \text{ gr}$$

7. Convert $\frac{1}{100}$ gr into metric weights.

   1 gr = 64.8 mg

   $$\frac{1}{100} \text{ gr} = 64.8 \times \frac{1}{100} = 0.648 \text{ mg}$$

8. Convert $\frac{1}{6}$ gr into mgs.

   1 gr = 64.8 mg

   $$\frac{1}{6} \text{ gr} = 64.8 \frac{1}{6} = 10.8 \text{ mg}$$

9. Convert 30 m into ml.

   16.23 m = 1 ml

$$1 \text{ m} = \frac{1}{16.23} \text{ ml}$$

$$30 \text{ m} = \frac{1}{16.23} \times 30 = 1.848 \text{ ml}$$

10. Convert 2 pt into ml.

    1 pt = 20 fl. oz

    2 pt = 20 × 2 = 40 fl. oz

    1 fl. oz = 29.57 ml

    40 fl. oz = 29.57 × 40 = 1182.8 ml

    2 pt = 1182.8 ml.

Calculations Based on Imperial Systems

For preparing 1% w/v solns any of the following formulas which are identical in strength can be used:

	I	II	III	IV
Solid	1 gr	4.375 gr	35 gr	1 oz (Avoir)
Solvent to produce	110 m	1 fl. oz	8 fl. oz	100 fl. oz

Formula I should be used when the volume of the solution required is small and the strength of such solution is weak. Formula II, III & IV may be used according to the quantities of the solutions to be prepared.

While using formula I it is important to note that it is not permitted to weigh less than 1 gr of solid on the dispensing balance because of its low sensitivity. Hence, the volume prepared may be much more than the required volume. The excess volume so prepared may be rejected or preserved for further prescriptions to be dispensed.

1. Rx

    Atropine sulphate   ½ %

    Aqua q.s.

Calculations

1 gr of atropine sulphate dissolved in 110 m = 1% W/V soln

1 gr of atropine sulphate dissolved in 220 m = ½ % W/V soln.

Dispense 120 m or 2 drachms out of the above soln and reject the remainder.

2. Prepare 1 oz of 1/8 % solution of zinc sulphate in equal volumes of normal saline solution and adrenaline solution.

Calculations

Since two solvents, i.e., normal saline solution and adrenaline solution are used out of which adrenaline solution is costlier than normal saline solution therefore dissolve zinc sulphate at double strength in normal saline solutions.

1 gr of zinc sulphate dissolved in 110 m of normal saline solution
$$= 1\% \text{ W/V soln}$$
1 gr of zinc sulphate dissolved in 440 m of normal saline solution
$$= 1/4 \% \text{ W/V soln}$$
Take out 240 m of the above solution and mix it with 240 m of adrenaline solution. The resulting 480 m (1 oz) solution will be 1/8%.

3. Prepare 4 oz of 5% solution of a substance.

Calculations

35 gr dissolved in 8 fl. oz = 1% W/V soln

35×5 gr dissolved in 8 fl. oz = 5% W/V soln

$\dfrac{35 \times 5}{8}$ gr dissolved in one fl. oz = 5% W/V soln

$\dfrac{35 \times 5 \times 4}{8} = 87.5$ gr dissolved in 4 fl. oz = 5% W/V soln

Therefore, weigh 87.5 gr of the substance and dissolve in sufficient amount of water to produce 4 fl. oz. The resulting solution will be 5% solution.

4. Send 1 pint of a 1 in 500 solution of potassium permanganate.

Calculations

35 gr of potassium permanganate dissolved in 8 fl. oz
$$= 1\% \text{ W/V soln}$$

$35 \times \dfrac{100}{500}$ gr of potassium permanganate dissolved in 8 fl. oz

$$= \frac{1}{5} \% \text{ W/V soln (1 in 500)}$$

$$\frac{35 \times 100 \times 500}{8} \text{ gr of potassium permanganate dissolved in one fl. oz}$$

$$= \frac{1}{5} \% \text{ W/V soln}$$

$$\frac{35 \times 100 \times 20}{500 \times 8} = 17.5 \text{ gr of potassium permanganate dissolved in}$$

$$20 \text{ fl. oz} = \frac{1}{5} \% \text{ W/V soln}$$

Therefore, weigh 17.5 gr of potassium permanganate and dissolve in sufficient amount of water to produce 1 pint. The resulting solution will be 1 in 500 solution.

5. How many tablets each containing 8.75 gr of mercuric chloride will be required to make one quart of 0.05% solution.

Calculations

35 gr dissolved in 8 fl. oz = 1% W/V soln

35×0.05 gr dissolved in 8 fl. oz = 0.05 % W/V soln

$$\frac{35 \times 0.05}{8} \text{ gr dissolved in one fl. oz} = 0.05\% \text{ W/V soln}$$

$$\frac{35 \times 0.05}{8} \times 40 = \frac{35 \times 5 \times 40}{8 \times 100} = 8.75 \text{ gr dissolved in 40 fl. oz}$$

$$= 0.05\% \text{ W/V soln}$$

8.75 gr of mercuric chloride contained in 1 tablet

1 gr of mercuric chloride contained in $\dfrac{1}{8.75}$ tablet

8.75 gr of mercuric chloride will be contained in $\dfrac{1}{8.75} \times 8.75$

$$= 1 \text{ tablet.}$$

Therefore, each tablet of 8.75 gr of mercuric chloride will make one quart of 0.05% solution.

Solutions dispensed in concentrated form

6. Required 6 oz of a solution so that 2 teaspoonfuls diluted to a pint will make a 1 in 1000 solution.

   This problem will be solved in two parts.

   (a) Calculate the no. of grains required to make one pint of a 1 in 1000 solution.

   (b) Every two teaspoonfuls of the concentrated solution must contain these number of grains. Therefore multiply these number of grains with the number of two teaspoonfuls contained in 6 oz.

(a) 35 gr dissolved in 8 fl. oz = 1 in 100 soln

$$\frac{35 \times 100}{1000} \text{ gr dissolved in 8 fl. oz} = 1 \text{ in } 1000 \text{ soln}$$

$$\frac{35 \times 100}{1000 \times 8} \text{ gr dissolved in one fl. oz} = 1 \text{ in } 1000 \text{ soln}$$

$$\frac{35 \times 100 \times 20}{1000 \times 8} = 8.75 \text{ gr dissolved in 20 fl. oz} = 1 \text{ in } 1000 \text{ soln.}$$

Therefore, 8.75 gr of the drug must be contained in every 2 teaspoonfuls of the solution.

(b) 6 oz = 6 × 8 = 48 teaspoonfuls
2 teaspoonfuls contain 8.75 gr

$$1 \text{ teaspoonful contains} = \frac{8.75}{2} \text{ gr}$$

$$48 \text{ teaspoonfuls must contain} \frac{8.75}{2} \times 48 = 210 \text{ gr.}$$

Therefore, dissolve 210 gr of the drug in water and dilute to 6 fl oz.

Sometimes concentrated solutions may be prescribed and the pharmacist is asked to label with directions to prepare weaker percentage solutions.

7. Send 4 oz of a 10% solution of potassium permanganate and label with directions for preparing a quart of a 1 in 400 solution.

Calculations

These types of problems are also calculated in two parts.

(a) Calculate the number of grains required to make 4 oz of a 10% solution.

(b) Calculate the quantity to be diluted to a quart to make a 1 in 400 solution.

(a) 35 gr dissolved 8 fl. oz = 1% W/V soln

35 × 10 gr dissolved in 8 fl. oz = 10% W/V soln

$$\frac{35 \times 10}{8} \text{ gr dissolved in one fl. oz} = 10\% \text{ W/V soln}$$

$$\frac{35 \times 10 \times 4}{8} = 175 \text{ gr dissolved in 4 fl. oz} = 10\% \text{ W/V soln.}$$

Therefore, dissolve 175 gr in water and dilute it to 4 fl. oz.

(b) A 10% solution means 1 in $\dfrac{100}{10}$ = 1 in 10 soln.

That is, 10 oz of the solution contains 1 oz of the substance

or, 10 oz of this solution diluted to 400 oz will produce 1 in 400 solution

or, $\dfrac{10 \times 40}{400}$ = 1 oz diluted to one quart will produce 1 in 400 solution.

Therefore, label with direction to dilute 1 oz or 2 tablespoonfuls to a quart.

EXERCISES (A)

Calculate the quantities required to prepare the following:

1. Atropine sulphate 1%. Send 4 drachms.
2. Acriflavine 0.1% in a mixture of equal volume of alcohol and water. Send 2 oz.
3. 8 oz of a 1 in 2000 solution.
4. 1 gallon of a 1 in 1000 solution.
5. 1 pint of a 0.01% solution.
6. 4 oz of a 0.625% solution.
7. 1 quart of a normal saline solution.

8. How many tablets each containing 8.75 gr of corrosive sublimate will be required to make 1 pint of a 0.4% solution.

9. 8 oz of a solution so that 1 tablespoonful to half a gallon makes 1 in 500 solution.

10. 8 oz so that 1 tablespoonful to half a gallon will make a 1 in 2000 solution.

11. 10 oz of a 2.5% solution and label with the directions for preparing a quart of 0.0625% solution.

12. 10 oz of 6% solution and label with the directions for preparing 30 oz of a 0.05% solution.

13. From 20% solution supplied prepare a quart of a 0.0625% solution.

14. From 8% solution supplied prepare 1 pint of a 1 in 1000 solution.

Calculations based on metric system

1. Calculate the formula for 40 gm coal tar and zinc ointment from the official formula given below:

Yellow soft paraffin	600 gm
Zinc oxide, finely sifted	300 gm
Strong coal tar solution	100 gm

Quantities required for 40 gm $= \dfrac{40}{1000} \times$ official quantities.

2. Calculate the formula for 250 ml of oily lotion of calamine from the formula given below:

Calamine	50 gm
Wool fat	10 gm
Oleic acid	5 ml
Arachis oil	500 ml

Calcium hydroxide solution sufficient to produce 1000 ml

Quantities required for 250 ml $= \dfrac{250}{1000} \times$ quantities given.

3. Rx

Hyoscine hydrobromide	0.6 mg

Make powders. Send such 10 powders.

Calculations

To get the required quantities for 10 powders, multiply the given quantity by 10.

4. *Rx*

Heavy magnesium carbonate	8.125	gm
Light magnesium carbonate	8.125	gm
Rhubarb, in powder	6.25	gm
Ginger, in powder	2.5	gm

Make powder. Send 100 gm.

Calculations

To get the required quantities for 100 gm, multiply the given quantities by 4.

Percentage Calculations

(i) *Weight in Volume (W/V) Solutions*

In this the solute is weighed and the solvent is measured. The general formula for 1% W/V solution is:

Solid	1 part by weight
Solvent to produce	100 parts by volume.

1 gm solute dissolved in sufficient amount of water to produce 100 ml or 10 mg in 1 ml of water makes 1% W/V solution.

Unless and until specially specified the solutions in pharmacy are supplied as W/V solutions.

(ii) *Weight in Weight (W/W) Solutions*

In this the solute and the solvent are taken by weight. The general formula for 1% W/W solution is:

Solid	1 part by weight
Solvent to produce	100 parts by weight.

Percentage solutions of solids in liquids are not made W/W unless specially requested.

(iii) *Volume by Volume (V/V) Solutions*

In this solute and the solvent are taken by volume. The general formula for 1% V/V solution is:

Solute	1 part by volume
Solvent to produce	100 parts by volume.

1 ml solute dissolved in sufficient amount of solvent to produce 100 ml.

5. Calculate the quantity of sodium chloride required to prepare 500 ml of a 2% solution.

Calculations

1 gm of sodium chloride dissolved in water to produce 100 ml

$$= 1\% \text{ W/V soln.}$$

1 × 2 gm of sodium chloride dissolved in water to produce 100 ml

$$= 2\% \text{ W/V soln.}$$

For 500 ml the quantity of sodium chloride required

$$= \frac{1 \times 2 \times 500}{100} = 10 \text{ gm.}$$

Therefore, dissolve 10 gm of sodium chloride in sufficient amount of water to produce 500 ml. The resulting solution will be 2% solution.

6. Calculate the quantity of sodium chloride required for preparing 200 ml of a 0.9% solution.

Calculations

1 gm of sodium chloride dissolved in water to produce 100 ml

$$= 1\% \text{ W/V soln.}$$

1 × 0.9 gm of sodium chloride dissolved in water to produce 100 ml

$$= 0.9\% \text{ W/V soln.}$$

For 200 ml the quantity of sodium chloride required

$$= \frac{1 \times 0.9 \times 200}{100} = 1.8 \text{ gm.}$$

Therefore, dissolve 1.8 gm of sodium chloride in sufficient amount of water to produce 200 ml. The resulting solution will be 0.9% solution.

7. Prepare 30 ml of 10% solution of methyl salicylate in alcohol.

Calculations

For 100 ml solution the quantity of methyl salicylate required

$$= 10 \text{ ml}$$

For 30 ml solution the quantity of methyl salicylate required

$$= \frac{10 \times 30}{100} = 3 \text{ ml.}$$

Therefore, mix 3 ml of methyl salicylate with sufficient alcohol to produce 30 ml. The resulting solution will be 10% solution.

8. Prepare 50 ml of 0.1% solution of acriflavine in a mixture of equal volume of alcohol and water.

Calculations

Alcohol is relatively expensive but water is inexpensive, therefore, prepare the acriflavine solution at double strength in water and then add alcohol.

Double the strength of 0.1% = 0.2%

1 gm of acriflavine dissolved in 100 ml of water = 1% W/V soln.

1 × 0.2 gm of acriflavine dissolved in 100 ml of water
$$= 0.2\% \text{ W/V soln.}$$

For 50 ml solution the quantity of acriflavine required

$$= \frac{1 \times 0.2 \times 50}{100} = 0.1 \text{ gm} = 100 \text{ mg.}$$

Therefore, dissolve 100 mg of acriflavine in 50 ml water. Out of this, measure 25 ml and mix it with 25 ml alcohol. The resulting solution will be 0.1% solution of acriflavine in a mixture of equal volume of alcohol and water.

9. Prepare 100 ml of a 1 in 4000 solution of potassium permanganate.

Calculations

$$1 \text{ in } 4000 = \frac{100}{4000} \text{ per cent} = 0.025\%$$

1 gm of potassium permanganate dissolved in 100 ml water
$$= 1\% \text{ W/V soln.}$$

1 × 0.025 gm of potassium permanganate dissolved in 100 ml water
$$= 0.025\% \text{ W/V soln.}$$

For 100 ml solution the quantity of potassium permanganate required

$$= \frac{1 \times 0.025 \times 100}{100} = 0.025 \text{ gm} = 25 \text{ mg.}$$

Therefore, dissolve 25 mg of potassium permanganate in sufficient water to produce 100 ml. The resulting solution will be 1 in 4000 solution.

10. Send 150 ml of 4% potassium permanganate solution and label with directions for preparing 500 ml of a 1 in 2500 solution.

Calculations

(a) 1 gm of potassium permanganate dissolved in 100 ml water

= 1% W/V soln.

1 × 4 gm of potassium permanganate dissolved in 100 ml water

= 4% W/V soln.

For 150 ml the quantity of potassium permanganate required

$$= \frac{1 \times 4 \times 150}{100} = 6 \text{ gm.}$$

Therefore, dissolve 6 gm of potassium permanganate in sufficient water to produce 150 ml solution.

(b) Strength of concentrated solution = 4%

Strength of dilute solution = 1 in 2500 = $\dfrac{100}{2500} = \dfrac{1}{25} = 0.04\%$

Degree of dilution = $\dfrac{4}{0.04} = 100$ times.

Quantity of concentrated solution required = $\dfrac{500}{100} = 5$ ml.

Therefore, dilute 5 ml of concentrated potassium permanganate soln upto 500 ml with water. The resulting solution will be 1 in 2500 solution.

11. From 1 in 400 solution of acriflavine, prepare 100 ml of 1 in 5000 solution.

Calculations

Strength of concentrated acriflavine soln provided

$$= 1 \text{ in } 400 = \frac{100}{400} = \frac{1}{4} = 0.25\%$$

Strength of dilute solution = 1 in 5000 = $\dfrac{100}{5000} = \dfrac{1}{50} = 0.02\%$

Degree of dilution = $\dfrac{0.25}{0.02} = \dfrac{25}{2}$ times.

Quantity of concentrated solution required = $\dfrac{100 \times 2}{25} = 8$ ml.

Therefore, dilute 8 ml of concentrated solution of acriflavine upto 100 ml with water. The resulting solution will be 1 in 5000 solution.

Alcohol Dilutions

Dilute alcohols are made from 95% alcohol which contains 95 parts ethyl alcohol and 5 parts water. All other dilutions of alcohol are prepared by mixing the specified parts of alcohol and water.

On mixing alcohol with water, contraction in volume and rise in temperature occurs and mixture becomes turbid. The turbidity is caused by minute air bubbles evolved from the alcohol on dilution. Because air is less soluble in water than in alcohol, so on addition of water air is partly expelled from the solution. Since there will be contraction in volume and rise in temperature, consequently it is necessary to cool the mixture to about 20°C before adjusting to the final volume.

The general formula for calculating the amount of stronger alcohol required to make a weaker alcohol is as under:

Volume of stronger alcohol to be used

$$= \frac{\text{volume required} \times \text{percentage required}}{\text{percentage used}}$$

12. Prepare 600 ml of 60% alcohol from 95% alcohol.

Calculations

Volume of 95% alcohol to be used $= \dfrac{600 \times 60}{95} = 379$ ml.

Therefore, take 379 ml of 95% alcohol, dilute it upto 600 ml with water. The resulting dilution will contain 60% alcohol.

13. Prepare 500 ml of 40% alcohol from 95% alcohol.

Calculations

Volume of 95% alcohol to be used $= \dfrac{500 \times 40}{95} = 210$ ml.

Therefore, dilute 210 ml of 95% alcohol upto 500 ml with water. The resulting dilution will contain 40% alcohol.

Weight in Weight (W/W) Solutions

The general formula is as under:

Weight of stronger acid to be used

$$= \frac{\text{weight required} \times \text{percentage required}}{\text{percentage used}}$$

14. Send 200 ml of a solution of acetic acid containing 4% of real acetic acid. The strength of real acetic acid is 33%.

    Calculations

    Weight of stronger acid to be used $= \dfrac{200 \times 4}{33} = 24.2$ gm.

    Therefore, weigh 24.2 gm of real acetic acid and dilute it upto 200 ml with water. The resulting solution will contain 4% acetic acid.

15. Send 200 ml of a solution of ammonia containing 4% by weight of ammonia. The strong solution of ammonia contains 32.5% of ammonia W/W.

    Calculations

    The weight of strong ammonia required $= \dfrac{200 \times 4}{32.5} = 24.615$ gm.

    Therefore, dilute 24.615 gm of strong solution of ammonia to 200 gm with water. The resulting solution will contain 4% ammonia.

Alligation Method

The calculations for exercises from 12 to 15 may be done by a method known as alligation method. This method is not recommended except as a method of checking because there are chances of errors in writing the figures.

16. Prepare 1000 gm of dilute acetic acid 4% from 33% real acetic acid.

    Calculations

    The weight of real acetic acid required $= \dfrac{1000 \times 4}{33} = 121.2$ gm

    The amount of water required $= 1000 - 121.2 = 878.8$ gm.

By alligation method

Subtract 0 (for water) from 4 = 4
Subtract 4 from 33 = 29
4 parts of real acetic acid and 29 parts of water will constitute 33
parts by weight of dilute acetic acid.

Therefore, the quantity of real acetic acid required

$$= \frac{1000 \times 4}{33} = 121.2 \text{ gm}$$

and the quantity of water required $= \dfrac{1000 \times 29}{33} = 878.8$ gm.

17. Prepare 400 ml of 70% alcohol from 95% alcohol.

Calculations

Volume of 95% alcohol to be used $= \dfrac{400 \times 70}{95} = 294.74$ ml

Volume of water to be used = 400 − 294.74 = 105.26 ml.

By alligation method

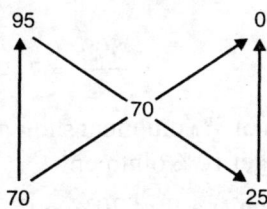

Subtract 0 (for water) from 70 = 70
Subtract 70 from 95 = 25
70 parts of 95% alcohol and 25 parts of water will constitute the
required % alcohol.

∴ quantity of 95% alcohol required $= \dfrac{400 \times 70}{95} = 294.74$ ml

and the quantity of water required $= \dfrac{400 \times 25}{95} = 105.26$ ml.

18. Find out the quantity of 3% ointment which must be added to 100 gm of a 15% ointment to get 10% ointment.

Calculations

By applying alligation rule

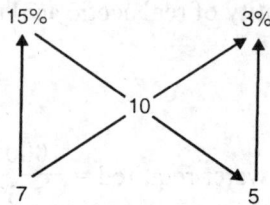

i.e., 7 parts of 15% ointment and 5 parts of 3% ointment must be mixed to get 10% ointment. The given strength of 100 gm ointment is 15%. So find out the relative proportion of 3% ointment required.

7 parts of 15% ointment require 5 parts of 3% ointment

1 part of 15% ointment requires $\dfrac{5}{7}$ parts of 3% ointment

100 parts of 15% ointment require $\dfrac{5}{7} \times 100$ parts of 3% ointment

$$= \frac{500}{7} = 71.43 \text{ gm of 3% ointment.}$$

Therefore, 71.43 gm of 3% ointment should be mixed with 100 gm of 15% ointment to get 10% ointment.

19. Find out that how many parts of 70%, 60%, 40% and 30% alcohol should be mixed to get 55% alcohol.

Calculations

By applying alligation rule

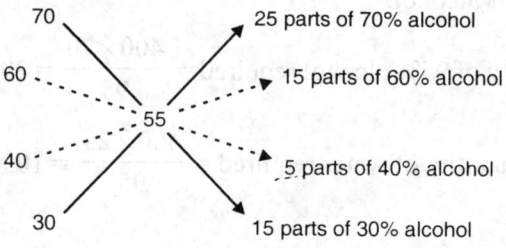

Therefore, when 25 parts of 70% alcohol, 15 parts of 60% alcohol, 5 parts of 40% alcohol and 15 parts of 30% alcohol are mixed together, the resulting solution will produce 55% alcohol.

Check:

(25 × 70) + (15 × 60) + (5 × 40) + (15 × 30)

$$= 1750 + 900 + 200 + 450 = 3300$$

(25 + 15 + 5 + 15) 55 = 60 × 55 = 3300.

20. Find out the amount of each of 90%, 60%, 30% and water required to produce 500 ml of 50% alcohol.

Calculations

By applying alligation rule

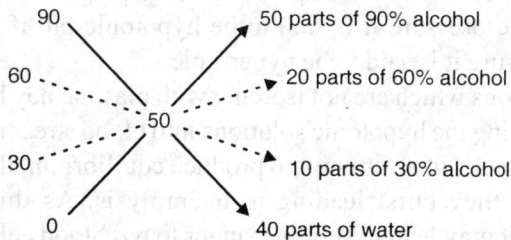

Therefore, when 50 parts of 90% alcohol, 20 parts of 60% alcohol, 10 parts of 30% alcohol and 40 parts of water are mixed together, the resulting solution will produce 50% alcohol.

Check:

(50 × 90) + (20 × 60) + (10 × 30) + (40 × 0)

$$= 4500 + 1200 + 300 + 0 = 6000$$

(50 + 20 + 10 + 40) 50 = 120 × 50 = 6000.

EXERCISES (B)

1. Prepare 500 ml of 1 in 5000 solution of potassium permanganate.
2. Send 100 ml of 2% acriflavine solution.
3. Supply 500 ml of normal saline solution.
4. Prepare 300 ml of 45% alcohol from 90% alcohol.
5. Prepare 400 ml of 55% alcohol from 95% alcohol.
6. Send 200 ml of 60% alcohol from 95% alcohol.
7. Supply 500 ml of 20% alcohol from 95% alcohol.
8. From 90% alcohol provided supply 400 ml of 60% alcohol.

9. From 60% alcohol supplied prepare 2 litres of 45% alcohol.
10. Supply 250 ml of solution containing 15% of real acetic acid. The strength of official acetic acid is 33.
11. Prepare 120 ml of solution containing 20% of real acetic acid. The real acetic acid is 33% W/W.
12. Prepare 1000 gm of 6% acetic acid from 33% acetic acid.

ISOTONIC SOLUTIONS

All the ophthalmic and injectable solutions should be isotonic, e.g., ophthalmic solutions should be isotonic with lachrymal secretions (tears) to prevent irritation and pain, similarly, injectable solutions should be isotonic with blood plasma. Solutions having the same osmotic pressure are said to be isotonic. As compared to blood plasma if a solution has lower osmotic pressure it is said to be hypotonic but if it has higher osmotic pressure it is said to be hypertonic.

The solutions which are not isotonic with plasma may be harmful to use. On injecting the hypotonic solutions into blood stream, it may enter the red blood cells in an attempt to produce equilibrium, the cells swell rapidly until they burst leading to haemolysis. As this damage is irreversible, it may lead to serious danger to red blood cells.

When hypertonic solution is injected into the blood stream, the water comes out of the membrane of red blood cells in order to reach equilibrium. The cells shrink leading to crenulation which is only a temporary damage. When the osmotic pressure of two solutions becomes equal, the damaged cells will come to their original position. Hence hypertonic solutions may therefore be administered without permanent damage to the blood cells. They should be injected slowly to ensure rapid dilution into the blood stream and to minimise the crenulation of blood cells.

For the adjustment of tonicity of injectable solutions, substances like sodium chloride and dextrose, etc., are added. About 0.9% solution of sodium chloride is isotonic, 0.45% solution is hypotonic and 5% solution of sodium chloride is hypertonic with plasma.

Proof Spirit

For excise purposes, the strengths of alcoholic preparations are indicated by degrees "over proof" (O.P.) or "under proof" (U.P.). Proof spirit is legally defined as that mixture of alcohol and water which at 51°F weighs

12/13th of an equal volume of water. In India and Britain, this standard is equal to 57.1% V/V or 49.28% W/W of ethyl alcohol. Such a spirit has a sp. gr. of 0.91976 at 15.5°C. Whereas in USA 50% V/V of ethyl alcohol is considered to be 100 proof.

Any alcoholic solution which contains 57.1% V/V alcohol is a proof spirit and is said to be 100 proof. Any strength above proof strength is expressed as over proof (O.P.) and any strength below proof strength is expressed as under proof (U.P.). In India the rates of excise duty are charged in terms of rupees per litre of proof alcohol.

Any % V/V of alcohol can be converted into proof strength and vice versa by using the following method:

Multiply the % strength of alcohol by 1.753 and deduct 100 from the product. If the result is positive it is known as over proof and if the result is negative then it is known as under proof.

The figure 1.753 is obtained as follows:

57.1 volumes of ethyl alcohol = 100 volume of proof spirit

$$1 \text{ volume of ethyl alcohol} = \frac{100}{57.1} = 1.753 \text{ volumes of proof spirit}$$

Example 1. Find the strength of 90% V/V alcohol in terms of proof spirit.

Applying the formula

90 volumes of ethyl alcohol = $90 \times 1.753 - 100 = 157.77 - 100$
$$= +57.77 \text{ or } 57.77° \text{ O.P.}$$

Example 2. Calculate the real strength of 40° O.P. and 50° U.P.

Applying the formula

40 over proof means $100 + 40 = 140$

$$\text{Alcohol strength} = \frac{140}{1.753} = 79.86\% \text{ V/V}$$

50 under proof means $100 - 50 = 50$

$$\text{Alcohol strength} = \frac{50}{1.753} = 28.52\% \text{ V/V}$$

Check if strength is 79.86% V/V and 28.52% V/V value of proof will be

(i) $79.86 \times 1.753 - 100 = 139.99 - 100 = + 39.99 \text{ or } 40° \text{ O.P.}$

(ii) $28.52 \times 1.753 - 100 = 49.99 - 100 = - 50.01 \text{ or } 50° \text{ U.P.}$

Example 3. A sample of brandy is 30 under proof. Calculate its alcoholic strength V/V.

30 under proof means $30 - 100 = 70$

$$\text{Alcoholic strength} = \frac{70}{1.753} = 39.93 \text{ or } 40\% \text{ V/V.}$$

Example 4. How many proof gallons are contained in 4 gallons of 70% V/V alcohol.

Applying the formula

Value of proof = % strength of alcohol × 1.753 – 100

$$= 70 \times 1.753 - 100 = 122.71 - 100$$
$$= +22.71 \text{ or } 22.71° \text{ O.P.}$$

That means

100 gallons of 70% V/V alcohol $= 100 + 22.71$

$$= 122.71 \text{ gallons of proof spirit}$$

$$1 \text{ gallon of 70\% V/V alcohol} = \frac{122.71}{100} \text{ gallons of proof spirit}$$

$$4 \text{ gallons of 70\% V/V alcohol} = \frac{122.71}{100} \times 4 \text{ gallons of proof spirit}$$

$$= 4.90 \text{ gallons of proof spirit}$$

Therefore, 4 gallons of 70% V/V alcohol are equivalent to 4.90 gallons of proof spirit.

EXERCISES (C)

1. Convert the following strength of alcohol into proof spirit:
   (i) 70.74% V/V   (ii) 50.16% V/V
   (iii) 25.78% V/V   (iv) 79.87% V/V
   (v) 47.31% V/V

2. Convert the following degree of proof spirit into % V/V strength of alcohol:
   (i) 44.6° O.P.   (ii) 18.4° O.P.
   (iii) 35.3° O.P.   (iv) 75.0° U.P.
   (v) 54.8° U.P.

3. How many proof gallons are represented by 50 wine gallons of 90% V/V alcohol.

ANSWERS

(A)

1. 3 gr of atropine sulphate to be dissolved in sufficient water to produce 330 m.
2. Take 1 gr acriflavine and dissolve it in sufficient water to produce 550 m. Out of this measure out 480 m and mix it with 480 m alcohol. Produce the final volume to 2 oz because there will be little contraction in volume which occurs when alcohol is diluted with water.
3. 1.750.   4. 70.0 gr.
5. 0.875 gr.   6. 10.9375 gr.
7. 157.5 gr.   8. 4 tablets.
9. 70 gr, 1120 gr.   10. 17.5 gr, 280 gr.
11. 109.375 gr, two tablespoonful to be diluted to a quart.
12. 262.5 gr, two teaspoonful to be diluted to 30 oz.
13. 1/8 oz or 60 minims. 14. 1/4 oz or 120 minims.

(B)

1. Dissolve 100 mg potassium permanganate in sufficient water to produce 500 ml solution.
2. Dissolve 2 gm acriflavine in sufficient water to produce 100 ml solution.
3. Dissolve 4.5 gm sodium chloride in sufficient water to produce 500 ml solution.
4. 150 ml.   5. 231.578 ml.
6. 126.315 ml.   7. 105.263 ml.
8. 266.666 ml.   9. 1.5 lit.
10. 113.636 gm.   11. 72.72 gm.
12. 181.818 gm.

(C)

1. (i) 24° O.P. (ii) 12.07° U.P. (iii) 54.81° U.P. (iv) 40° O.P. (v) 17.07° U.P.
2. (i) 82.48% V/V (ii) 67.54% V/V (iii) 77.18% V/V (iv) 14.26% V/V (v) 25.78% V/V.
3. 78.88 proof gallons.

Posology

The word posology is derived from the Greek words 'posos', meaning how much and 'logos', meaning science. That means it is a branch of medical science which deals with doses or quantity of drugs which can be administered to produce the required pharmacological actions.

The dose of a drug may be defined as the quantity of drug which is "enough but not, too much," the idea is to produce the drug's optimum therapeutic effect in a particular patient with the lowest possible dose. The pharmacopoeias and textbooks usually give a minimum and maximum dose for each drug. Minimum dose is necessary to produce a desired therapeutic effect but maximum dose is the largest quantity which can be given safely to an individual without producing harmful effects. Beyond the maximum dose certain toxic effects and undesirable effects may be produced.

The dose of a drug cannot be fixed rigidly because there are so many factors which influence the doses, e.g., age, condition of the patient, severity of the disease, natural tolerance, acquired tolerance, idiosyncrasy, route of administration, degree of absorption and rate of elimination. The doses listed below are not binding upon the prescriber, considering the above mentioned factors he can change the doses accordingly.

The doses mentioned in the table represent the average maximum quantities of drugs which can be administered to an adult orally within 24 hours; when other routes of administration are followed the relevant appropriate dose is mentioned. If the doses are to be administered in divided doses, the frequencies of administration are stated.

The doses given here are for general guidance. It is the responsibility of the prescriber regarding the amount of drug prescribed or the frequency at which the drug is administered. But before dispensing any medication it is the duty of the pharmacist to satisfy himself that overdose has not been prescribed. In case of doubt he should consult the prescriber and to confirm the doses of individual medicaments he can consult the extra pharmacopoeia.

DOSES PROPORTIONATE TO AGE

Calculation of Child Dose

The dose for a child from adult dose can be calculated by any one of the following formulas:

(A) According to Age

1. Young's Rule

$$\text{Child's dose} = \frac{\text{age in years}}{\text{age in years} + 12} \times \text{adult dose}$$

For example, if the adult dose is 60 mg and the age of the child is 4 years, the dose for the child will be

$$\frac{4}{4 + 12} \times 60 = \frac{4}{16} \times 60 = \frac{1}{4} \times 60 = 15 \text{ mg}$$

2. Dilling's Rule

$$\text{Child's dose} = \frac{\text{age in years}}{20} \times \text{adult dose}$$

For example, if the adult dose is 60 mg and the age of the child is 6 years, the dose for the child will be

$$\frac{6}{20} \times 60 = \frac{3}{10} \times 60 = 18 \text{ mg}$$

Because of quicker and easy calculations, Dilling's rule is considered better.

3. Clark's Formula (according to body weight)

$$\text{Child's dose} = \frac{\text{child's weight (kg)}}{70} \times \text{adult dose}$$

For example, if the adult dose is 60 mg and the weight of the child is 14 kg, the dose for the child will be

$$\frac{14}{70} \times 60 = 12 \text{ mg}$$

DOSES PROPORTIONATE TO SURFACE AREA

The calculation of child's dose according to surface area is more appropriate rather than the methods based on age. This method is more complicated than the methods based on age but tables have been provided by which dose for a child can be calculated. This methods is based on the following formula:

$$\frac{\text{Surface area of child} \times 100}{\text{Surface area of adult}} = \text{Percentage of adult dose}$$

Table

Age	Percentage of adult dose
One month	10
2 months	15
4 months	20
1 year	25
3 years	35
5 years	40
10 years	60
12 years	75
16 years	90

FACTORS AFFECTING DOSE AND ACTION OF DRUGS

Various factors which influence the dose and action of a drug in an individual are as follows:

1. Age

In determining the dose of a drug the age of an individual is of great significance specially in the young or very old persons. Children and old persons need lesser amount of drug than the standard adult dose because they are unable to inactivate or excrete drugs to that extent as adults but at the same time children can tolerate relatively large doses of digitalis and belladonna on the basis of their body weights as compared with adults. Newborn infants are abnormally sensitive to certain drugs because of the immature state of their hepatic and renal function by which drugs are normally inactivated and eliminated from the body.

2. Body Weight

Generally recommended adult doses are based on a "normal" body weight of 70 kg. But such a dose will be too less for a muscular person weighing 100 kg and too large for a weak person weighing about 50 kg. The calculation of doses for children on the basis of body weight is considered more dependable than that based strictly on age. The doses calculated according to body weight are expressed as mg/kg body weight.

3. Sex

Generally females require lesser dose than males because of their lesser weight and also due to the reason that they are more responsive to the effects of certain drugs than males. Drugs should be given very carefully during menstruation, pregnancy and lactation. Strong purgatives should be avoided during menstruation, whereas drugs which stimulate contraction of uterus should be avoided in pregnant ladies which may lead to abortion or miscarriage. Drugs like alcohol, anaesthetic gases, barbiturates, narcotic and non-narcotic analgesics, etc., which are readily transported from mother to the foetal circulation should be avoided. These drugs produce adverse effects to the foetus sometimes resulting in death of the foetus in the uterus. During lactation, drugs such as antihistaminics, morphine and tetracyclines which are excreted in milk should be given very cautiously to the mothers who are breast-feeding the babies.

4. Route of Administration

The dose of a given drug may vary according to the dosage form and route of administration used. Drugs administered intravenously enter the blood stream directly hence require lesser dose than the subcutaneous dose which in turn is smaller than the oral dose.

5. Time of Administration

Time of administration of drugs is very important. Drugs are rapidly absorbed from the empty stomach, hence an amount of drug that is effective when taken before a meal may be ineffective if administered during or after meals. On the other hand irritating drugs are better tolerated if administered after meals which will dilute the drug's concentration and reduce the gastric irritation, e.g., iron, arsenic, cod-liver oil, etc., should always be given on a full stomach.

6. Presence of Disease

Drugs are more effective in diseased conditions than normal body conditions. During fever one can tolerate high doses of antipyretics than in a nonfebrile condition. Similarly during hepatic or renal disturbances, the drugs which are metabolised in the liver or excreted through the kidneys may prove fatal.

7. Environmental Factors

Alcohol is better tolerated in cold environments than in summer. Dose of a sedative required to produce sleep during day time is much more than the dose required to produce sleep during night.

8. Emotional Factors

Females are more emotional and responsive to drugs therefore require less dose of drugs. The faith inspired by the doctor on the mind of a patient is an important factor in medication. Nervous patients require smaller doses of drugs as compared to normal patients.

9. Accumulation

When a drug is repeatedly administered for a long time, depending on its nature, it may unexpectedly accumulate in the body to produce sudden toxic symptoms. The drugs which produce such symptoms of poisoning are called cumulative drugs. The cumulative effects are usually produced by slow excretion, defective degradation or unexpectedly rapid absorption of drugs. Therefore drugs like digitalis, emetine, bromides, heavy metals should be carefully administered but cumulative effect is desirable in drugs like chloroquin and phenobarbitone which are used in cases of malaria and epilepsy respectively.

10. Synergism

When two or more drugs are used in the combined form their action is either increased or decreased depending on the drugs used in combination. When the potency or duration of action is increased, the phenomenon is called synergism. This synergism is of two types: (a) addition and (b) potentiation.

(a) Addition

When the total effect of two drugs is just equal to the sum of their individual effects, it is known as addition.

(b) Potentiation

When the combined effect of two drugs administered is greater than the sum of their individual effects, it is known as potentiation, e.g., combination of ephedrine and adrenaline acts as a better bronchodialator.

Synergism is very useful where desired therapeutic result needed is difficult to obtain with a single drug especially if single drug produces side effects. By this action dose of individual drugs can be lowered.

11. Antagonism

When the action of one drug is opposed by the other drug, the phenomenon is known as antagonism. The total combined effect is less than the algebraic total effect of the two drugs, e.g., milk of magnesia is given in acid poisoning. Here one drug is acidic and another is alkaline. They react with each other or in other words it may be said that the effect of one drug is antagonised by the other drug. Similarly if adrenaline and acetylcholine are given together they neutralise the effect of each other because adrenaline is vasoconstrictor whereas acetylcholine is vasodilator.

12. Habituation and Addiction

(a) Habituation

When repeated use of a drug or agent leads to production of emotional or psychological dependence rather than compulsion the condition is known as habituation, e.g., use of tea, coffee, tobacco, chewing of betel nut, tranquilizers, etc. When such agents are withdrawn the individual can carry on his routine work. Here there is no physical dependence, hence it can be easily tackled.

(b) Addiction

It is a state of psychic and physical drug dependence. Continuous use of alcohol, opium, cocaine, heroin, morphine, pethidine, LSD leads to addiction and turns the person to a wreck who becomes liability to society. The addicts are deeply attached to the drug and become slave of it, therefore craves for it at all times and tries to procure it by any means, fair or foul. If he is unable to get the drug, he develops withdrawal symptoms which may be serious enough to produce death. So the drugs which lead to addiction must be prescribed very cautiously.

13. Idiosyncrasy

All persons do not respond alike to the same drug due to varied individual susceptibility, some may produce abnormal reaction to a drug. When an abnormal or unusual reaction is produced by a drug it is known as idiosyncrasy, e.g., few mg of aspirin may produce gastric haemorrhage and small doses of quinine may produce ringing in the ear.

14. Hypersensitivity

Hypersensitivity is an allergic reaction to a drug and is different from either the expected pharmacological response or toxic reaction to the drug. This is due to frequent or indiscriminate use of drugs like antibiotics, vitamins and especially proteinous substances. Once a person is sensitised, a minute dose of the drug will produce allergic reactions. It is of two types (i) immediate type which is serious and requires prompt injection of adrenaline otherwise death may occur (ii) delayed type in which urticaria, skin rashes or contact dermatitis may occur.

15. Tolerance

When a drug administered in an ordinary dose fails to produce the normal therapeutic effect and requires large dose of the drug to produce the normal effect. The unusual resistance thus produced is known as tolerance, e.g., smokers can tolerate nicotine, alcoholics can tolerate large doses of alcohol, rabbits can tolerate large doses of atropine due to quick destruction of the drug by enzyme atropine estrase present in their blood.

TACHYPHYLAXIS

It is also known as acute tolerance. It is observed in certain drugs that when they are administered repeatedly at very short intervals the cell receptors get blocked up and pharmacological response to that particular drug is decreased. By increasing the dose this decreased response cannot be reversed. But if the administration of the drug is stopped for a long time and administered again after being discontinued then the initial effect of the drug can be reobserved. This condition is known as tachyphylaxis. Drugs like ephedrine, amphetamine, cocaine, and nitrites behave in this way.

Doses of Different Drugs, their Route of Administration and Uses

Name of drug	Maximum doses	Route of administration	Uses
Adrenaline acid tartrate	0.4 to 1 mg	By s/c injection as single dose	Sympathomimetic
Adrenaline injection	0.2 to 0.5 ml	By s/c injection as single dose	Sympathomimetic
Aluminium hydroxide gel	7.5 to 15 ml	Oral	Antacid
Dried aluminium hydroxide gel	0.5 to 1 gm	Oral	Antacid
Aminophylline	100 to 300 mg	Oral	Bronchodialator
	250 to 500 mg	By slow i/v injection	
Amphetamine sulphate	5 to 20 mg	Oral, daily in divided doses	Central nervous system stimulant
Ampicillin	1 to 6 gm	Oral, daily in divided doses	Antibiotic
Amylobarbitone	100 to 200 mg	Oral	Hypnotic
Amylobarbitone sodium	400 mg	Oral, daily in divided doses	Sedative
Aneurine hydrochloride (Vit. B_1)	5 mg	Oral, daily prophylactic dose	Vitamin B_1 deficiency
	100 mg	Oral, daily therapeutic dose	Vitamin B_1 deficiency
	100 mg	By s/c or i/m injection	Vitamin B_1 deficiency
Antazoline hydrochloride	100 to 300 mg	Oral, daily in divided doses	Antihistaminic
Apomorphine hydrochloride	2 to 8 mg	By s/c or i/m injection	As an emetic
Ascorbic acid (Vit. C)	25 to 75 mg	Oral, prophylactic dose	For preventing scurvy
	250 mg	Oral, therapeutic dose	For treating scurvy

(Contd.)

Name of drug	Maximum doses	Route of administration	Uses
Aspirin (Acetyl salicylic acid)	0.3 to 1 gm	Oral	Analgesic and antipyretic
	4 to 8 gm	Oral, daily in divided doses	In the treatment of acute rheumatism
Atrophine sulphate	0.25 to 2 mg	Oral, daily in single or divided doses	Parasympatholytic
	0.25 to 2 mg	By s/c, i/m or i/v injection	Parasympatholytic
BCG vaccine	0.1 ml	By intracutaneous injection as prophylactic dose	Active immunisation against tuberculosis
Barbitone sodium	300 to 600 mg	Oral	As hypnotic
	900 mg	Oral, daily in divided doses	As sedative
Belladonna dry extract	15 to 60 mg	Oral	Antispasmodic
Belladonna tincture	0.5 to 2 ml	Oral	Antispasmodic
Bemegride	1 gm	50 mg repeated at an interval of ten minutes by i/v injection according to the need of the patient	In the treatment of barbiturate poisoning
Benzylpenicillin	0.5 to 3 gm	Oral, daily in divided doses	Antibiotic
	0.3 to 6 gm	By i/m or i/v injection daily in divided doses	Antibiotic
Butobarbitone	100 to 200 mg	Oral	Hypnotic
Caffeine	100 to 300 mg	Oral	Central nervous system stimulant
Caffeine citrate	100 to 300 mg	Oral	Central nervous system stimulant

(Contd.)

Name of drug	Maximum doses	Route of administration	Uses
Calciferol	20 mcg	Oral	In the prevention of rickets
	0.125 to 1.25 mg	Oral	In the treatment of rickets and osteomalacia
Calcium carbonate	1 to 5 gm	Oral	Antacid
Calcium gluconate	1 to 5 gm	Oral	In the treatment of calcium deficiency
	1 to 2 gm	By i/m or i/v injection	
Calcium lactate	1 to 5 gm	Oral	In the treatment of calcium deficiency
Castor oil	5 to 20 ml	Oral	Cathartic purgative
Chloral hydrate	0.3 to 2 gm	Oral	Hypnotic
Chloramphenicol	1.5 to 3 gm	Oral, daily in divided doses	Antibiotic
Chlordiazepoxide	10 to 100 mg	Oral, daily in divided doses	Tranquilizer
Chloroform spirit	0.25 to 2 ml	Oral	Flavour and preservative
Chloroquin phosphate	500 mg	Oral, weekly	In suppression of malaria
	0.5 to 1.5 gm	Oral, daily	In the treatment of malaria
	200 to 300 mg (base)	By i/m or i/v injection	In the treatment of malaria
	0.5 to 1 gm	Oral, daily in divided doses	In the treatment of hepatic amoebiasis
Chlorothiazide	0.5 to 2 gm	Oral	Diuretic

(Contd.)

Name of drug	Maximum doses	Route of administration	Uses
Chlorpheniramine maleate	4 to 16 mg	Oral, daily in divided doses	Antihistaminic
	5 to 20 mg	By i/m injection as a single dose	
Chlorpromazine hydrochloride	75 to 800 mg	Oral, daily in divided doses	In psychiatric states
	25 to 50 mg	Oral and by i/m injection	As an antiemetic
Chlortetracycline hydrochloride	1 to 3 gm	Oral, daily in divided doses	Antibiotic
Codeine phosphate	10 to 60 mg	Oral	In cough and diarrhoea; also acts as weak analgesic
Cod liver oil	10ml	Oral	In the prevention of rickets
Cortisone acetate	50 to 400 mg	Oral and by i/m injection daily in divided doses	Corticosteroid
Cyanocobalamin (Vit. B_{12})	1 mg	Initial dose by i/m injection repeated ten times at intervals of two or three days	In the treatment of vitamin B_{12} deficiency and in the treatment of megaloblastic anaemia
	250 mcg	Maintenance dose by i/m injection every four weeks until the blood count is normal	In the treatment of vitamin B_{12} deficiency and in the treatment of megaloblastic anaemia
Dexamethasone	10 mg	Oral, daily in divided doses	Corticosteroid
Diazepam	5 to 30 mg	Oral, daily in divided doses	Tranquilizer
	5 to 10 mg	By i/m or slow i/v injection	

(Contd.)

Name of drug	Maximum doses	Route of administration	Uses
Digoxin	1.5 mg	Initial dose, in single or divided doses, for rapid digitalisation	In the treatment of congestive heart failure
	50 mcg	Maintenance dose, daily	
Di-iodohydroxy-quinoline	1 to 2.0 gm	Oral, daily in divided doses	In the treatment of amoebiasis
Emetine hydrochloride	30 to 60 mg	By s/c or i/m injection daily	In the treatment of amoebiasis
Ephedrine hydrochloride	15 to 60 mg	Oral	In the treatment of asthma
Ergometrine maleate	0.5 to 1 mg	Oral and by i/m injection	Uterine stimulant
Ergotamine tartrate	1 to 2 mg	Oral	In the treatment of migraine
	250 to 500 mcg	By s/c or i/m injection	
Erythromycin	1 to 4 gm	Oral, daily in divided doses	Antibiotic
Erythromycin estolate	≡ 1 to 4 gm base	Oral, daily in divided doses for not more than 10 days	Antibiotic
Ferric ammonium citrate	1 to 6 gm	Oral, daily in divided doses	In the prevention and treatment of iron deficiency anaemia
Ferrous sulphate	300 mg	Oral, daily prophylactic dose	In the prevention and treatment of iron deficiency anaemia
	900 mg	Oral, in divided doses, daily therapeutic dose	In the treatment of iron deficiency anaemia

(Contd.)

Name of drug	Maximum doses	Route of administration	Uses
Folic acid	5 to 20 mg	Oral, daily	In the treatment of megaloblastic anaemia
	200 to 500 mcg	Oral, daily	In prophylaxis of megaloblastic anaemia of pregnancy
Frusemide	40 to 120 mg	Oral	Diuretic
Gentamycin sulphate	80,000 to 240,000 units	By i/m injection daily, in divided doses	Antibiotic
Griseofulvin	0.5 to 1 gm	Oral, daily in divided doses	Antifungal-antibiotic
Halibut liver oil	0.2 to 0.5 ml	Oral	Source of vitamin A
Heparin	10,000 to 15,000 units	By i/v or i/m injection	Anticoagulant
Hydrocortisone acetate	5 to 50 mg	By intra-articular injection	Corticosteroid
Hyoscine hydrobromide	300 to 600 mcg	Oral and by s/c injection	Central nervous system depressant and also used in motion sickness
Hyoscyamus tincture	2 to 5 ml	Oral	Central nervous system depressant and also used in motion sickness
Ipecacuanha liquid extract	0.1 ml	Oral	Expectorant and emetic
Ipecacuanha tincture	1 ml	Oral	Expectorant and emetic

(Contd.)

Name of drug	Maximum doses	Route of administration	Uses
Isoniazid	300 to 600 mg	Oral, daily in divided doses	Used in tuberculosis along with streptomycin
Light kaolin	15 to 75 gm	Oral	Antidiarrhoeal; antacid
Liquid extract of liquorice	2 to 5 ml	Oral	Expectorant
Light and heavy magnesium carbonate	250 to 500 mg	Oral	As an antacid
	2 to 5 gm	Oral	As a laxative
Light magnesium oxide	250 to 500 mg	Oral	As an antacid
	2 to 5 gm	Oral	As a laxative
Liquid paraffin	10 to 30 ml	Oral	As a laxative
Magnesium hydroxide mixture	5 to 10 ml	Oral	As an antacid
	25 to 50 ml	Oral	As a laxative
Magnesium sulphate	15 gm	Oral	Purgative
Magnesium trisilicate	0.5 to 2 gm	Oral	As an antacid
Male fern extract	3 to 6 ml	Oral	In threadworm infestation
Meprobamate	0.4 to 1.2 gm	Oral, daily in divided doses	Sedative
Methyldopa	≡ 0.5 to 3 gm anhydrous methyldopa	Oral, daily in divided doses	In the treatment of hypertension
Morphine hydrochloride	10 to 20 mg	Oral	Narcotic analgesic
Morphine sulphate	10 to 20 mg	Oral, by s/c or i/v injection	Narcotic analgesic
Nalorphine hydrobromide	5 to 10 mg	Initial dose by i/v injection; repeated in accordance with patient's needs to a total dose not exceeding 40 mg	Antidote for morphine poisoning

(Contd.)

Name of drug	Maximum doses	Route of administration	Uses
Neomycin sulphate	1.4 to 4.2 mega units	Daily, in divided doses	As an intestinal antiseptic
Nicotinamide	15 to 30 mg	Oral, prophylactic	A component of vitamin B complex
	50 to 250 mg	Oral, daily therapeutic dose	
Nicotinic acid	15 to 30 mg	Oral, prophylactic dose	A component of vitamin B complex
	50 to 250 mg	Oral, daily therapeutic dose	
Nikethamide	0.5 to 2 gm	By i/v injection	Respiratory stimulant
Noscapine	15 to 30 mg	Oral	Cough suppressant
Nux vomica liquid extract	0.05 to 0.2 ml	Oral	Bitter tonic
Nux vomica tincture	0.5 to 2 ml	Oral	Bitter tonic
Nystatin	1 to 2 mega units	Oral, daily in divided doses	Antifungal antibiotic
Oxyphenbutazone	200 to 400 mg	Oral, daily in divided doses	Analgesic and anti-inflammatory
Oxytetracycline hydrochloride	1 to 3 gm	Oral, daily in divided doses	Antibiotic
Paracetamol	0.5 to 1 gm	Oral	Analgesic, antipyretic
	up to 4 gm	Oral, daily in divided doses	
Paraldehyde	5 to 10 ml	Oral and by i/m injection	Hypnotic, sedative, anti-convulsant
	15 to 30 ml	By rectal injection	As a basal anaesthetic

(Contd.)

Name of drug	Maximum doses	Route of administration	Uses
Pentobarbitone sodium	100 to 200 mg	Oral	Hypnotic
Peppermint oil	0.05 to 0.2 ml	Oral	Carminative and flavouring agent
Pethidine hydrochloride	50 to 100 mg	Oral and by s/c and i/m injection	Narcotic analgesic
	50 mg	By i/v injection	
Phenacetin	300 to 600 mg	Oral	Analgesic and antipyretic
Phenobarbitone	up to 350 mg	Oral, in divided doses	Hypnotic, anti-convulsant
Phenobarbitone sodium	up to 350 mg	Oral, in divided doses	Hypnotic, anti-convulsant
Phenolphthalein	50 to 300 mg	Oral	Laxative
Phenoxymethyl-penicillin	0.5 to 1.5 gm	Oral, daily in divided doses	Antibiotic
Phenylbutazone	200 to 400 mg	Oral, daily in divided doses	Analgesic and anti-inflammatory
Phthalylsulphathiazole	5 to 10 gm	Oral, daily in divided doses	Antibacterial agent used in large intestine
Piperazine citrate	1 to 2 gm	Oral, daily in divided doses	In the treatment of threadworm infestation
Piperazine phosphate	4.5 gm	Oral, single dose	In the treatment of roundworm infestation
Potassium bromide	1 to 6 gm	Oral, daily in divided doses	Sedative
Potassium iodide	250 to 500 mg	Oral	As an expectorant
	150 mg	Oral, daily in divided doses	In the preoperative treatment of thyrotoxicosis

(Contd.)

Name of drug	Maximum doses	Route of administration	Uses
Prednisolone	5 to 60 mg	Oral, daily in divided doses	Corticosteroid
Prednisone	5 to 60 mg	Oral, daily in divided doses	Corticosteroid
Primaquin phosphate	≡ 15 mg base	Oral, daily for 14 days	In the cure of malaria
Procaine penicillin	300 to 900 mg	Daily by i/m injection	Antibiotic
Progesterone	20 to 60 mg	Daily by i/m injection	Progestational steroid
Pseudoephedrine hydrochloride	60 to 180 mg	Oral, daily in divided doses	Used for the relief of nasal congestion
Pyridoxine hydrochloride (Vit. B_6)	100 to 300 mg	Oral, daily in divided doses	A component of vitamin B complex
Quinine hydrochloride	300 to 600 mg	Oral, daily	In suppression of malaria
Quinine sulphate	1.2 to 2 gm	Oral, daily in divided doses	In the treatment of malaria
Reserpine	1 to 5 mg	Oral, daily in divided doses	In psychiatric states
	100 to 500 mcg	Oral, daily	In the treatment of hypertension
Riboflavine (Vit. B_2)	1 to 4 mg	Oral, prophylactic dose	A component of vitamin B complex
Smallpox vaccine	5 to 10 mg	Oral, daily therapeutic dose	In prevention of smallpox
	0.02 ml	Prophylactic dose by scarification or pressure inoculation	
Sodium bicarbonate	1 to 5 gm	Oral	As an antacid
Sodium bromide	1 to 6 gm	Oral, daily in divided doses	Sedative

(Contd.)

Name of drug	Maximum doses	Route of administration	Uses
Sodium citrate	up to 10 gm	Oral, daily in divided doses	Systemic alkalinising substance
Sodium iodide	250 to 500 mg	Oral	As an expectorant
	150 mg	Oral, daily in divided doses	In the preoperative treatment of thyrotoxicosis
Sodium salicylate	5 to 10 gm	Oral, daily in divided doses	In the treatment of acute rheumatism
Streptomycin sulphate	≡ 500 mg base	Oral, every eight hours	As an intestinal antiseptic
	≡ 1 gm base	By i/m injection daily or at longer intervals	
Sulphadiazine	3 gm	Oral, initial dose subsequent doses up to 4 gm daily in divided doses	A sulphonamide used in the treatment of systemic infections
Sulphadimidine	3 gm	Initial dose, subsequent doses up to 6 gm daily in divided doses	A sulphonamide used in the treatment of systemic infections
	2 gm	Initial dose, subsequent doses up to 4 gm daily in divided doses	In the treatment of urinary infections
Testosterone	100 to 600 mg	By implantation	Anabolic steroid
Tetracycline hydrochloride	1 to 3 gm	Oral, daily in divided doses	Broad spectrum antibiotic

(Contd.)

Name of drug	Maximum doses	Route of administration	Uses
Thiamine hydrochloride (Vit. B₁)	2 to 5 mg	Oral, prophylactic dose	A component of vitamin B complex
	25 to 100 mg	Oral, daily therapeutic dose	
	25 to 100 mg	By s/c or i/m injection	
Thyroid	30 to 250 mg	Oral, daily	In hypothyroidism
Tolbutamide	0.5 to 1.5 gm	Oral, daily	In the treatment of mild diabetes
Vasopressin injection	0.25 to 0.75 ml (5 to 15 units)	By s/c or i/m injection	In the treatment of diabetes
Viomycin sulphate	0.5 to 1 mega unit	By i/m injection daily or at longer intervals	Antibiotic

IMPORTANT INSTRUCTIONS FOR COMMONLY USED DRUGS

The following instructions or directions given by the physician or the pharmacist must be followed by the patient or his attendant which must be complied with. Noncompliance of these directions may lead to serious consequences. The correct advice in a very simple language help the patient to a great extent. Some common examples are given below:

Drug	Instructions
1. Salicylates	Do not take on an empty stomach.
2. Antacid tablets	These must be chewed and not to be swallowed.
3. Antidiabetics	Avoid consumption of alcoholic beverages.
4. Ampicillin	It should be taken one hour before or two hours after food.
5. Bisacodyl (Dulcolax)	Do not take antacid or milk within one hour of taking the drug.
6. Diazepam (may lead to drowsiness)	1. Do not drive a vehicle which requires full alertness. 2. Do not work with dangerous machinery. 3. Do not drink alcohol/alcoholic beverages.
7. Diphenylhydramine (causes sedation)	Do not drive the vehicle.
8. Liquid paraffin (lubricant laxative)	It must not be used for prolonged time.
9. Phenylbutazone and oxyphenylbutazone	Do not take on an empty stomach.
10. Tetracyclines	Do not take with milk.

CHAPTER
5

Pharmaceutical Incompatibilities

A pharmaceutical incompatibility may be defined as the result of prescribing or mixing the substances which are antagonistic in nature and an undesirable product is formed which may affect the safety, purpose or appearance of the preparation. These incompatibilities are of three general types, i.e., physical, chemical and therapeutic.

Physical incompatibilities are those when two or more than two substances are combined together, a physical change takes place and an unacceptable product is formed. Since these changes which take place are usually visible therefore they can be easily corrected by applying the pharmaceutical skill to obtain an acceptable preparation.

Chemical incompatibilities are those in which a chemical reaction takes place between the ingredients and a new undesirable compound is formed. These types of incompatibilities are little difficult to correct and in some cases it may be necessary to eliminate or substitute one of the reacting substances, dispense them in separate containers, change them to non- reactive form or to pack and store in suitable containers. In such cases the physician should be consulted and informed.

THERAPEUTIC INCOMPATIBILITY

Therapeutic incompatibility may be the result of prescribing certain drugs to the patient with the intention to produce a specific degree of action but the nature or the intensity of the action produced is different from that intended by the prescriber. It may be due to the administration of (i) overdose or improper dose of a single drug; (ii) wrong dose or dosage form; (iii) contraindicated drugs; (iv) synergistic and antagonistic drugs.

Rx

Codeine phosphate   0.6 gm
Make powders. Send such 10 powders.
Type: Therapeutic incompatibility.

In the present prescription an overdose of codeine phosphate has been prescribed. Therefore the prescription must be referred back to the prescriber.

Rx

Tetracycline hydrochloride   250 mg
Make capsules. Send such 10 capsules.
Label: Take one capsule every six hours with milk.
Type: Therapeutic incompatibility.

In this prescription the direction is wrong. Tetracycline is inactivated by calcium which is present in milk. Therefore tetracycline capsules should not be taken with milk. Hence refer back the prescription to the prescriber for the directions to be changed.

Although the physician is responsible for the prescribed medications but the pharmacist must be aware of the possibility of errors and whenever he finds some error in the prescription, he must consult the prescriber for the correct dispensing of prescription. This will save the prescriber, the pharmacist and the patient from serious consequences.

Incompatibilities of physical and chemical type may be either instantaneous or delayed. In the first case visual changes like effervescence, liquefaction or precipitation may take place. In the delayed incompatibilities the reaction or changes take place at a later stage, e.g., crystallization, cracking of emulsions or colour change, etc.

Now a days the prescriptions are generally written for the official and proprietary preparations which are prepared by the pharmaceutical industries and are available in pharmaceutical prepackaged form. Rarely the prescriptions are compounded by the pharmacist but even then the pharmacist must be conversant with the incompatibilities which take place in compounding the pharmaceutical preparations. By applying the pharmaceutical, chemical and pharmacological background he must decide the most suitable line of action to get the desired product.

PHYSICAL INCOMPATIBILITY

Physical incompatibility is usually due to immiscibility, insolubility, precipitate formation or liquefaction of solid materials. This usually causes non-uniform, unsightly or unpalatable mixtures. Sometimes it becomes very difficult to measure an accurate dose from non-uniform products. Usually these types of difficulties can be easily overcome by applying the pharmaceutical skill to present the product with the best possible appearance and to ensure uniform doses of medication. Generally physical incompatibilities may be corrected by one or more of the following method, i.e., order of mixing, alteration of solvents, change in the form of ingredients, alteration of volume, emulsification, addition of suspending agent; addition, substitution or omission of therapeutically inactive substances to facilitate the compounding of the prescription.

Examples of Physical Incompatibilities and Their Methods of Correction

1. Oils and water are immiscible with each other. They can be made miscible by emulsification, e.g., castor oil emulsion, olive oil emulsion, liquid paraffin emulsion, etc.

   Rx

Olive oil	30 ml
Water	up to 120 ml

   Make an emulsion.

   Type: Physical incompatibility.

   In this prescription olive oil (a fixed oil) is immiscible with water. To make them miscible, an emulsifying agent will have to be incorporated.

2. In liquid preparations containing indiffusible solids such as prepared chalk, acetyl salicylic acid, succinyl sulphathiazole, sulphadimidine, phenacetin, zinc oxide and calamine, etc., a suspending agent will have to be incorporated so as to increase the thickness of the preparation and to maintain uniform distribution of the substances for sufficiently long time after shaking the bottle thus facilitating uniform measurement of each dose.

Rx

Phenacetin	3 gm
caffeine	1 gm
Orange syrup	12 ml
Water	up to 90 ml

Make a mixture.

In this prescription phenacetin is an indiffusible substance, so to make it diffusible a suspending agent, either compound tragacanth powder or tragacanth mucilage, will have to be used.

3. Certain powders like sulphur, antibiotics and certain corticosteroids are insoluble in water and are difficult to wet with water. Some wetting agents like saponins or polysorbates may be used to distribute these powders in water.

4. Resins are insoluble in water, therefore when a resinous tincture is added to water the resin forms indiffusible clots which can be prevented either by slowly adding the undiluted tincture with vigorous stirring to the diluted suspension, or by adding some suitable thickening agent.

5. Oils dissolved in alcohol separate out on the addition of water.

6. High concentrations of electrolytes cause cracking of soap emulsions by salting out the emulsifying agent.

7. Addition of a common solvent in an emulsion which may dissolve the oily phase, the aqueous phase and the emulsifying agent lead to the formation of one phase system, e.g., addition of alcohol in turpentine liniment.

8. Certain low melting point solids, when mixed together liquefy due to the formation of eutectic mixtures. Substances when any two of them are mixed together liquefy or form a soft mass include camphor, menthol, thymol, phenol, chloral hydrate, sodium salicylate, acetyl salicylic acid and phenazone.

These types of substances create problem when they are to be dispensed in powder form. For this purpose they can either be triturated together to form liquid and mixed with an absorbent like light kaolin or light magnesium carbonate to give a free flowing product or each ingredient is powdered separately and mixed with an absorbent and then combined together lightly and filled in suitable containers.

Rx

Menthol	5 gm
Camphor	5 gm
Ammonium chloride	30 gm
Light magnesium carbonate	60 gm

Make an insufflation.

Type: Physical incompatibility.

In the above prescription, menthol, camphor and ammonium chloride are liquefiable substances. When any two of them are combined together they liquefy and form a eutectic mixture. Therefore to dispense them in powders light magnesium carbonate is added which acts as an absorbent.

CHEMICAL INCOMPATIBILITY

Chemical incompatibility may be result of chemical interactions between the ingredients of a prescription and a harmful or even dangerous product may be formed. Therefore precautions should be taken either to prevent the formation of harmful product or to correct them. In such cases the prescriber must be informed.

Generally chemical incompatibilities result from oxidation reduction, acid-base, hydrolysis or combination reactions. These reactions may be noticed by precipitation, effervescence, decomposition, colour change or by explosion and usually occur immediately when the prescription ingredients are mixed and thus these types of incompatibilities are called immediate incompatibilities. They should be dispensed only after correction. Sometimes the reactions proceed at a very slow rate and no appreciable visible change occurs which may develop on standing. Such types of incompatibilities are known as delayed incompatibilities. These types of incompatibilities may or may not result in loss of therapeutic activities.

Types of Chemical Incompatibilities

The chemical incompatibilities fall into two groups:

(a) Tolerated

In tolerated incompatibilities, where practicable the reaction is minimised by applying some suitable order of mixing or mixing the solutions in dilute forms but no alteration is made in the active ingredients of the preparation.

(b) Adjusted

In adjusted incompatibilities the reaction is prevented by addition or substitution of one of the reacting substances with another of equal therapeutic value but does not affect the medicinal action of the preparation (e.g., substitution of caffeine citrate with caffeine in sodium salicylate and caffeine citrate mixtures).

The incompatibility may be (i) intentional when the prescriber knowingly prescribes the incompatible drugs or (ii) it may be un-intentional when the prescriber prescribes the drugs without knowing that there is incompatibility in the prescribed drugs.

General Methods for Precipitate Yielding Combinations

Generally, it is noticed that reaction between strong solutions proceed at a faster rate and the precipitates formed are thick and do not diffuse readily whereas the reaction between the dilute solutions proceed at a slow rate and the precipitates formed are light and diffuse readily in the solution. Hence the reacting substances should be diluted to the maximum extent before mixing them. The precipitates so formed may be diffusible or indiffusible. The methods adopted for dispensing such prescriptions in which diffusible or indiffusible precipitates are formed will be described under the heading method A and method B.

Method A

This method is used when diffusible precipitates are formed and in those cases where the amount of precipitates formed is very small.

Divide the vehicle into two equal portions. Dissolve one of the reacting substances in one portion and the other in the other portion. Mix the two portions by slowly adding one portion to the other with rapid stirring.

Method B

This method is used when the indiffusible precipitates are formed and they form an appreciable portion of the mixture.

Divide the vehicle into two equal portions. Dissolve one of the reacting substances in one portion. Place the other portion of the vehicle in a mortar, to this incorporate a suitable amount of compound tragacanth powder (10 grains per ounce or 2 gm per 100 ml of the finished product) with constant trituration until a smooth mucilage is produced, then add and dissolve the other reacting substances. Mix the two portions by slowly adding one portion to the other with rapid stirring.

Whether method A or method B has been used in dispensing the prescription, it is very important to fix a "Shake the bottle." label to the container and ensure that the patient strictly follows and realises the importance of these directions.

METHODS OF CORRECTING CHEMICAL INCOMPATIBILITIES

1. Alkaloidal Salts with Alkaline Substances

Most alkaloidal salts are soluble in water but alkaloidal bases are practically insoluble in water and are freely soluble in organic solvents.

When an alkaline substance like aromatic spirit of ammonia, solution of ammonia, ammonium bicarbonate, sodium bicarbonate, potassium bicarbonate, borax, etc., is added to an alkaloidal salt solution the free alkaloid may be precipitated. However they are not always precipitated, because all alkaloids are slightly soluble in water and other added substances as for example:

(a) Strychnine

Tincture nux vomica is generally used as a source of strychnine in mixtures required to stimulate the appetite. The amount of strychnine present is 0.125 gm per 100 ml of tincture nux vomica and the solubility of strychnine is about 1 in 7000, i.e., 100 ml of water will dissolve

$$\frac{1 \times 100}{7000} = 0.143 \text{ gm of strychnine.}$$

Hence the amount of strychnine present in 10 ml of tincture nux vomica will be easily dissolved in 100 ml of water and will not be precipitated in alkaline solutions. Further, tinctures contain certain amount of alcohol due to which the precipitation is further prevented. Moreover the solubility of strychnine is much more in alcohol (i.e., 1 in 150) than in water. Therefore it follows that in mixtures containing sufficient amount of alcohol strychnine will not be precipitated even when more than 10 ml of tincture per 100 ml is present in the prescription.

Rx

Strychnine hydrochloride solution   6 ml
Aromatic spirit of ammonia   4 ml
Water   120 ml
Make a mixture.

Type: Chemical incompatibility (incompatibility of alkaloidal salts with alkaline substances).

Strychnine hydrochloride is an alkaloidal salt and aromatic spirit of ammonia is an alkaline substance. When they react together the precipitates of strychnine are formed because the quantity of strychnine hydrochloride prescribed is much more than its solubility, moreover the amount of alcohol present in aromatic spirit of ammonia is also negligible, hence strychnine gets precipitated. The precipitates so formed are diffusible in nature. Therefore follow method A for precipitate-yielding combinations.

(b) Morphine

The solubility of morphine is 12 minim per ounce. Therefore, preparations containing less than 12 minim per ounce of morphine will not be precipitated with alkaline substances. Further, morphine is more soluble in alcohol (i.e., 1 in 100) than in water. Therefore, in mixtures containing sufficient alcohol morphine will not be precipitated even if more than 12 minim per ounce is prescribed along with alkaline substances.

(c) Solanaceous Alkaloids

Tincture belladonna, tincture hyoscyamus and tincture stramonium containing solanaceous alkaloids are generally prescribed in mixtures, and the contents of these alkaloids in the prescribed amount is very low therefore are not precipitated in the alkaline solutions. Moreover presence of alcohol in tinctures further decreases precipitation.

(d) Ipecacuanha Alkaloids

Tincture ipecacuanha which contains emetine is mainly used in cough mixtures which may also contain alkaline substances like sodium bicarbonate or ammonium bicarbonate but emetine is not precipitated because the quality of tincture prescribed is very low and presence of alcohol further prevents precipitation.

(e) Codeine

Codeine is soluble in 120 parts of water or 2 parts of alcohol, because of its appreciable solubility in water the codeine is not precipitated from dilute solutions of its salts when mixed with alkaline substances.

(f) Caffeine

Caffeine is soluble in 80 parts of water or 40 parts of alcohol. It will not be precipitated in the doses prescribed in the prescriptions.

(g) Cocaine

Cocaine is slightly soluble in water (i.e., 1 in 1300) but fairly soluble in alcohol (1 in 10). Cocaine hydrochloride is generally used in eye drops, nasal sprays and throat sprays. In the presence of alkaline substances cocaine is precipitated therefore such formulations should not be dispensed. Cocaine eye drops must be dispensed in alkali-free containers.

(h) Quinine

Quinine is slightly soluble in water but very soluble in alcohol. Quinine is generally precipitated in mixtures when a normal dose of soluble quinine salt is prescribed with an alkaline substance so it should not be dispensed. However powders containing quinine and acetyl salicylic acid can be dispensed and used safely but they should not be kept and stored for a long time because darkening, and decomposition may take place, in which case they should be discarded.

2. Alkaloidal Salts with Soluble Iodides

Potassium iodide is generally prescribed as an expectorant in some of the cough mixtures also containing alkaloids but the quantity of alkaloids present (e.g., emetine from ipecacuanha tincture) is usually so low that the precipitation of hydriodide is unlikely to take place.

Strychnine when combined with soluble iodides forms a very insoluble hydriodide, the precipitates of which are diffusible hence follow method A for precipitate-yielding combinations.

3. Alkaloidal Salts with Tannins

When an alkaloidal salt is combined with a drug containing tannins, the alkaloids form tannates which are insoluble in water and the precipitates so formed are usually diffusible in nature therefore follow method A for precipitate-yielding combinations.

Since most alkaloids form insoluble tannates therefore this fact is frequently used in the treatment of alkaloidal poisoning in which case a strong solution of tannic acid or strong tea is administered which will precipitate the alkaloid and render it less harmful.

4. Alkaloidal Salts with Salicylates

Generally quinine compounds are prescribed with salicylates in the treatment of malaria. When quinine is combined with salicylates it forms indiffusible precipitates of quinine salicylate therefore follow method B for precipitate-yielding combinations.

Rx

Quinine hydrochloride	130 mg
Sodium salicylate	4 gm
Water	up to 90 ml

Make a mixture.

Type: Chemical incompatibility (incompatibility of alkaloidal salts with salicylates).

Quinine hydrochloride reacts with sodium salicylate to form the precipitates of quinine salicylate which are indiffusible in nature. Therefore follow method B for precipitate-yielding combinations.

Rx

Sodium salicylate	1.0 gm
Caffeine citrate	0.650 gm
Water	up to 30.0 ml

Make draught.

Type: Chemical (adjusted) incompatibility.

Caffeine citrate is a mixture of equal weights of caffeine and citric acid. The citric acid present reacts with sodium salicylate to liberate salicylic acid which gets precipitated. But if caffeine is used instead of caffeine citrate, it forms a soluble complex with sodium salicylate. Therefore substitute half as much caffeine as that of caffeine citrate and a clear mixture will be obtained.

5. Soluble Salicylates with Alkali Bicarbonates

When sodium salicylate is administered orally, it reacts with hydrochloric acid present in the stomach, liberating salicylic acid which is precipitated and leads to irritation of the gastric mucosa and pain in the stomach. Hence when sodium salicylate is prescribed it is usually given along with double the quantity of sodium bicarbonate as that of sodium salicylate, thereby partially neutralising the gastric secretion and thus minimising the formation and precipitation of salicylic acid.

When sodium salicylate is dispensed in the solution form, especially along with an alkaline substance like sodium bicarbonate the mixture absorbs oxygen from the atmosphere and becomes reddish brown in colour. This change does not significantly affect the therapeutic effectiveness of the medicament but may lead to confusion in the mind of the patient that the medicament has spoiled and he may not like to take it, therefore to avoid this confusion a colouring agent like liquid extract of liquorice or extract of burnt sugar may be added to darken the above mentioned mixture. If this is not done, the patient should be warned about the colour change. The colour change can also be retarded by adding an antioxidant such as sodium metabisulphite 0.1 percent but this should be added with the permission of the prescriber.

Rx

Sodium salicylate	1.0 gm
Sodium bicarbonate	1.0 gm
Sodium metabisulphite	0.01 gm
Chloroform water	up to 15.0 ml
Fiat mistura.	

Type: Simple mixture.

When sodium salicylate comes in contact with hydrochloric acid present in stomach, salicylic acid is formed which gets precipitated and leads to irritation in the stomach. Hence when sodium salicylate is prescribed it is usually prescribed with sodium bicarbonate which will temporarily neutralise the gastric secretion and thus minimise the formation of salicylic acid.

Sodium salicylate in solution form, specially when it is alkaline in nature, absorbs oxygen and solution becomes brownish black. Though the therapeutic value is not changed but it may lead to confusion in the mind of the patient that the mixture has spoiled and he may not like to use the mixture. Therefore to prevent the air oxidation, sodium metabisulphite is used as an antioxidant which will considerably retard the change in colour.

6. Soluble Salicylates and Benzoates with Acids

Most of the acids and acid syrups like syrup lemon B.P.C. which contain citric acid decompose sodium salicylate and sodium benzoate with the formation and precipitation of salicylic acid and benzoic acid respectively. The precipitates so formed are indiffusible in nature therefore follow method B for precipitate-yielding combinations. Otherwise syrup lemon which contains citric acid can be replaced (with the permission of the prescriber) without altering the therapeutic action of the preparation, with simple syrup and tincture lemon.

Rx

Sodium salicylate	5 gm
Syrup of lemon	20 ml
Water	up to 75 ml

Make a mixture.

Type: Chemical (adjusted) incompatibility.

Syrup of lemon contains citric acid. When it reacts with sodium salicylate, salicylic acid is formed which gets precipitated; the precipitates of which are indiffusible in nature.

Syrup of lemon is prescribed as a flavouring agent which can be replaced without altering the therapeutic action of the preparation. Therefore replace syrup of lemon with 19 ml of simple syrup and 1.2 ml of tincture of lemon.

7. Soluble Salicylates with Ferric Salts

Ferric salts react with sodium salicylate with the formation of precipitates of ferric salicylate which are indiffusible in nature. Therefore follow method B for precipitate-yielding combinations. In the presence of sodium bicarbonate the precipitates of ferric salicylate remain soluble therefore a clear mixture is obtained.

Rx

Ferric chloride solution	2 ml
Sodium salicylate	4 gm
Water	up to 90 ml

Make a mixture.

Type: Chemical incompatibility (incompatibility of salicylates with ferric salts).

Ferric chloride reacts with sodium salicylate to form ferric salicylate, the precipitates of which are indiffusible in nature. Hence follow method B for precipitate-yielding combinations.

8. Potassium Chlorate with Oxidisable Substances

When potassium chlorate is prescribed with an oxidisable substances like tannic acid, sugar, sulphur or any other readily oxidisable substance and heated or triturated together, there are chances of explosion. Therefore these dry substances should not be triturated together. They should be powdered separately in a dry and clean mortar and then mixed together lightly with a bone spatula on a paper or ointment slab without any friction.

9. Incompatibilities Causing Evolution of a Gas

When carbonates or bicarbonates are dispensed in the presence of an acid or acidic drug, they react together with the evolution of carbon dioxide. If the reaction is not allowed to complete and the mixture is transferred immediately to the bottle and corked there are chances of explosion with bursting of the bottle.

To prevent explosion, mix the ingredients in an open vessel and allow the reaction to complete until effervescence ceases. When whole of the carbon dioxide goes out, transfer the mixture to the bottle and cork. In some cases where the reaction proceeds slowly hot vehicle should be used to hasten the reaction.

(a) Borax with Sodium Bicarbonate and Glycerin

When borax and glycerin are mixed together, hydrolysis of borax takes place with the formation of sodium metaborate and boric acid. The boric acid so formed reacts with glycerin to form monobasic glyceryl boric acid. Boric acid itself is a weak acid therefore will not react with carbonates or bicarbonates whereas monobasic glyceryl boric acid formed is sufficiently strong to react with bicarbonates to liberate carbon dioxide.

When these three substances are to be compounded they should be mixed in an open vessel and mixture should not be transferred to the bottle until effervescence ceases. Hot water should be used as vehicle to hasten the reaction.

Rx

Sodium bicarbonate	1.5 gm
Borax	1.5 gm
Phenol	0.75 gm
Glycerin	25.00 gm
Water	up to 100.00 ml

Make a spray solution.

Type: Chemical incompatibility (incompatibility of evolution of carbon dioxide).

When sodium bicarbonate, borax and glycerin are mixed together in the presence of water, a reaction takes place with the evolution of carbon dioxide. If the mixture is dispensed as such, there are chances of bursting the bottle. Therefore mix these substances in an open vessel until evolution of carbon dioxide ceases. Incorporate phenol and transfer the mixture to the bottle.

(b) Bismuth Subnitrate and Sodium Bicarbonate

In the presence of water bismuth subnitrate reacts with sodium bicarbonate liberating carbon dioxide. This reaction proceeds slowly at ordinary temperature, hence the reaction should be accelerated by using hot water and mixture should not be transferred to the bottle until the effervescence ceases.

(c) Sodium Bicarbonate with Soluble Calcium or Magnesium Salts

When sodium bicarbonate is combined with soluble calcium or magnesium salts, double decomposition reaction takes place with the formation of corresponding insoluble carbonate and carbon dioxide. The precipitates of carbonates formed are diffusible in nature, so follow method A for precipitate-yielding combinations.

At ordinary temperature the reaction proceeds slowly, hence it should be accelerated by using the vehicle hot and mixture should not be bottled until effervescence ceases.

10. Liquid Extract of Liquorice in Acid Media

Liquid extract of liquorice has its flavouring properties due to the presence of glycyrrhizin, which is a sweet substance consisting of calcium and potassium salts of glycyrrhizinic acid. When liquid extract of liquorice is used as a flavouring agent in acid mixtures, the acid reacts with glycyrrhizin forming glycyrrhizinic acid which is precipitated and a sticky black sediment is formed which is difficult to diffuse. With the precipitation of glycyrrhizinic acid the flavouring property of the liquid extract is destroyed therefore it should not be used as flavouring agent in acid mixtures and should be used only in neutral or alkaline solutions. If prescribed in acid mixtures, the prescription should be referred back to the prescriber for substitution of a suitable flavouring agent.

11. Soluble Barbiturates with Ammonium Bromide

When soluble barbitone or soluble phenobarbitone is combined with ammonium bromide in the presence of water, a reaction takes place with the formation of barbitone which is insoluble in water therefore precipitated and precipitates so formed are indiffusible in nature, hence follow method B for precipitate-yielding combinations.

When soluble phenobarbitone is prescribed with ammonium bromide, it can be assumed that the prescriber intends the patient to receive a clear mixture, which can be produced by replacing chemically equivalent amount of ammonium bromide with sodium bromide or potassium bromide. Since the qualitative action of these bromides is the same, i.e., they produce sedative action therefore ammonium bromide can be replaced with sodium bromide or potassium bromide to get a clear mixture.

Rx

Phenobarbitone sodium	650 mg
Ammonium bromide	8 gm
Water	up to 120 ml

Make a mixture.

Type: Chemical incompatibility (incompatibility of soluble barbiturates with ammonium bromide).

In this prescription phenobarbitone sodium reacts with ammonium bromide with the formation of indiffusible precipitates of phenobarbitone. But if ammonium bromide is replaced with an equivalent amount of either sodium bromide or potassium bromide, a clear mixture is obtained. The pharmacological action of these three bromides is the same, but the intensity of action depends on the amount of bromide radicals used.

$$NH_4Br = NaBr$$
$$98 = 103$$

(mol. wt. of NH_4Br = 98, mol. wt. of NaBr = 103)

For 98 gm of NH_4Br the amount of NaBr required = 103 gm

For 1 gm of NH_4Br the amount of NaBr required = $\dfrac{103}{98}$ gm

For 8 gm of NH_4Br the amount of NaBr required = $\dfrac{103}{98} \times 8$ gm = 8.4 gm.

Therefore replace 8 gm of ammonium bromide with 8.4 gm of sodium bromide and prepare the mixture as such. The resulting mixture will be a clear mixture.

CHAPTER 6

Definitions and General Dispensing Procedures

Dispensing is an art and science of preparation and supply of medicaments to the users. Dispensing requires an extensive knowledge regarding
- stability of medicines and other substances of the prescription;
- principles of compounding;
- type of dosage form;
- incompatibilities i.e. chemical, physical and therapeutic;
- method of packaging and type of container, etc.;
- lebelling of the container, storage, supply and expiry date, etc.

GENERAL DISPENSING PROCEDURES

1. Work independently to avoid confusion and misunderstanding. Most of the retail pharmacies in majority of the countries is controlled and handled by one pharmacist who is a registered pharmacist and must be confident about the work he is going to do because he is to take many strong decisions himself. One should not hesitate to learn or to get knowledge from fellow pharmacists. If possible, such discussions should be done collectively in the classroom which will prove very useful and helpful.

2. Wear a freshly laundered white apron which not only protects your clothes but also reduces contamination of dispensed products with fibres and other particles. A coat is preferred than a jacket.

Wearing a well-laundered apron gives a professional look which creates a good impression in the mind of the patient and general public. Therefore, wear a spotlessly clean overall specially while working in the dispensary or drug store.

3. Keep a clean glass cloth, a duster, swab or sponge. These items will be used to polish the container before giving it to the patient. It will be unwise to use this glass cloth for wiping the bench/table. For cleaning the bench, table duster should be used which must be kept dry and a swab or sponge used to mop up wet spillage.

4. Work very carefully in a clean and tidy manner in order to reduce the risk of errors and contamination.

5. Do not accumulate the stock bottles and used apparatus in the working area. They must be replaced back on the same place from where they were taken.

6. Read the prescription carefully and be sure that it is understood by you. No guesswork of anything be done. In doubt, the prescriber or fellow pharmacists may be consulted to clear the things.

7. If necessary, find the correct formula from an appropriate source of information and note down the same in your practical notebook.

8. Check the doses of internal preparation from official books.

9. If any ingredient in the prescription has poisoning effect its weight/volume must be thoroughly checked and confirmed.

10. Be sure that there are no pharmaceutical incompatibilities.

11. Correct method of preparation must be understood. In case of doubt, fellow pharmacists may be consulted.

12. Proper storage conditions must be transferred to the label of the container.

13. Calculations regarding the ingredients of prescription must be worked out.

14. Label of the container must be read three times i.e. (i) while working out from the shelf, (ii) while weighing the contents (at this stage the label must be kept in the upward position to avoid spoilage of the label), and (iii) while keeping the containers back on the shelf.

15. Select the correct container and closure.

16. See that the label is appropriate to the container. It must not be too small or too big. If it is big, trim off properly.

17. Prepare the label and see that all the necessary instructions are written on the label.
18. Prepare the preparation, filter, if necessary.
19. Transfer the preparation to the required container.
20. Polish the container with a swab or glass cloth.
21. Label the container.
22. Make appropriate record in the notebook.

IMPORTANT INSTRUCTIONS

1. Do not light your burner with adjacent burner or by means of paper or stick.
2. Put off your burner when it is not in use.
3. Do not put off your burner with your mouth. It may lead to an accident.
4. Do not throw broken articles or burnt paper in the wash basin. For this always use dustbin.
5. Gas leakage, if any, must be reported immediately to the concerned person i.e. laboratory technician.
6. In case of a major accident, leave the laboratory and consult a doctor. In case of a minor accident, contact your teacher for first aid box.
7. Do not carry costly things to the laboratory.
8. While leaving the laboratory clean your working table with detergent and clean dry cloth.
9. Clean your hands with soap and water thoroughly.

7

Types of Dispensed Products
(Pharmacopoeial Preparations)

The following are short descriptions of pharmaceutical dosage forms and preparations that may be dispensed in the hospital pharmacy or on the retail counter.

AEROSOLS

The term aerosol has a specific meaning denoting a fine dispersion of liquid or solid particles in a gas where the particle size is less than 50 mm in diameter, as in the case of mist or smoke.

Aerosols may be defined as the pressurised dosage form of medicament in which the liquid or solid drug or drugs are dissolved or suspended in gas. The gas used for this purpose is known as propellant. The aerosols are packed in a suitable container known as aerosol container. When pressure is applied to the aerosol system, the contents are expelled out through the opening of the valve in the form of mist, a coarse, wet or dry spray, a stream or as a foam. The aerosols used in the treatment of respiratory conditions are atomised in devices known as atomisers or nebulisers. The type of atomiser used depends upon the viscosity of the spray solution; the more viscous the solution, the more powerful the atomiser needed.

Nowadays pharmaceutical aerosols are frequently used both orally and topically to dispense a large number of drugs including local analgesics, antiseptics, fungicidal agents, antibiotics and anti-inflammatory agents, etc. A number of veterinary and pet products have also been put into aerosol dosage forms. A variety of non-pharmaceutical preparations such as personal deodorant sprays, cosmetic hair sprays, perfume sprays, shaving lathers, tooth paste and various household products such as spray, starch, waxes, polishes, cleansers and lubricants are available as aerosols.

The potent drugs used for the relief of asthma are dissolved or suspended in a suitable solvent or propellant and are enclosed in a container which is fitted with a metering device that delivers a measured dose. Drugs administered in this way give rapid response and quick onset of action as compared with drugs administered orally. But the frequent use of such inhalations or sprays are not without risk and adverse reactions. Therefore it is advisable to warn the patient to strictly follow the directions given by the doctor and frequent use of such preparations should be avoided.

Aerosol containers provide a number of advantages over the more traditional methods of presentation of drugs that they are compact, convenient to carry and easy to apply evenly without touching the painful surfaces. A measured amount of drug and uniform doses are administered by metered valves. The product remains free from contamination and sterility of the preparation is maintained as no microorganisms can enter the pack when the valve is opened. They also provide good protection from oxidation and light to those drugs which are destroyed by air and light. Hydrolysis of drugs is prevented since the propellants contain no water. Because the filling and sealing of pressurised aerosols require special machinery and techniques therefore these preparations are costlier than traditional dosage forms.

APPLICATIONS

Applications are liquid or viscous preparations intended for application to the skin. Usually, they are suspensions or emulsions. Most of the official preparations contain parasiticides and are intended for only a limited number of applications. They should be dispensed in coloured fluted bottles in order to distinguish them from preparations meant for internal use. The container should be labelled "For external use only". Examples of applications are calamine application compound, B.P.C., dicophane application, B.P.C.

AROMATIC WATERS

Aromatic waters are also known as medicated waters. They are dilute, usually saturated, aqueous solutions of volatile oils or volatile substances. Some of them have a mild therapeutic action but mainly they are used as flavouring agents in preparations meant for internal administration of drugs. Aromatic waters may be prepared either by diluting the concentrated waters or by shaking the volatile substances with water. Aromatic waters include anise water, camphor water, chloroform water, cinnamon water and peppermint water.

CACHETS

Cachets consist of a dry powder enclosed in a shell, usually prepared from a mixture of rice flour and water by moulding into a suitable shape and drying. They are quite useful for administering the drugs with unpleasant taste and a large dose can be enclosed in a cachet than in a tablet or capsule.

There are two kinds of cachets; 'wet seal' cachets which are sealed by moistening the edges with water, and 'dry seal' cachets.

Before administration a cachet should be immersed in water for a few seconds, then placed on the tongue and swallowed with a draught of water. Cachets should be stored and supplied in well closed air-tight containers. Examples are sodium aminosalicylate cachets, sodium aminosalicylate and isoniazid cachets.

CAPSULES

Capsules are the solid unit dosage form of medicament in which the drug or drugs are enclosed in a practically tasteless, hard or soft soluble container or shell made up of a suitable form of gelatin. Hard capsules are used for filling the solid substances. Hard gelatin capsules are available in a number of sizes which varies from 000 to 5, the former being the largest and latter the smallest. They are made up of two cylindrical halves, one slightly larger in diameter but shorter in length known as cap and the other slightly shorter in diameter but longer in length know as base. The medicament is filled in longer narrower half, then the cap is fitted over the open end by moistening edges of the lower half of the capsule.

Soft capsules are flexible in nature. They may be spherical, ovoid, cylindrical or tubes. The spherical capsules are also known as 'Pearls'.

Soft gelatin capsules are used for enclosing the solids, liquids and semi-liquids.

Enteric coated capsules are the capsules which are treated or coated in such a way that the capsule does not disintegrate in the acidic medium of the stomach but disintegrates in the alkaline medium of the small intestine. Enteric coated capsules have been largely replaced by enteric coated tablets.

Capsules are increasing their popularity day by day. Hard capsule comes second to tablets in importance as solid unit dosage forms. Some of the capsules are administered through rectum and vagina and are convenient mode of administration of drugs than suppositories. For oral administration the capsule is placed on the tongue and swallowed with a drink of water.

COLLODIONS

Collodions are the liquid preparations meant for external application to the skin. They are convenient applications for small cuts and abrasions and are also used when a prolonged contact between the skin and the medicament is required. The vehicle used is volatile and evaporates on application to skin, leaving a flexible, protective film covering at the site of application. They are applied with a brush or rod.

Flexible collodion contains pyroxillon, castor oil and alcohol in solvent ether. Alcohol and solvent ether are used as vehicle, pyroxillon as film producing agent and castor oil gives flexibility.

CREAMS

Creams are viscous semisolid emulsions intended for application to the skin. Creams differ from ointments that they have lighter body than ointments. Moreover due to the presence of water soluble bases they can be easily removed from skin and clothings. Creams may be of oil in water (aqueous creams) or water in oil (oily creams) type. The aqueous creams have a tendency to bacterial and mold growth, therefore a preservative must be added in their formulation. Examples are cetomacrogol cream, cetrimide cream, chlorhexidine cream, hydrocortisone cream, etc.

DRAUGHTS (HAUSTUS)

A draught is a liquid oral preparation taken as a single dose. If several doses are prescribed, each dose is dispensed in separate container.

Ipecacuanha Emetic Draught, Paediatric is an exception where several doses are prescribed in a multipledose container. Examples are male fern extract draught and paraldehyde draught.

DUSTING POWDERS

Dusting powders are meant for external application to the skin. They are usually mixtures of two or more than two ingredients in fine powder e.g. starch, kaolin, talc, zinc oxide, etc. They must be homogeneous and in a very fine state of subdivision to enhance effectiveness and minimise local irritation. For this purpose they may be passed through sieve No. 120. Dusting powders are applied to the skin for antiseptic, antipruritic, astringent, antiperspirant, absorbent, protective and lubricant purposes.

Dusting powders are dispensed in sifter-top containers or pressure aerosols. They may also be supplied in wide mouth containers and applied with powder puff, a soft brush or a sterile gauge pad but care must be taken to avoid mechanical irritation to the skin surface. Dusting powders should not be applied to open wounds or to raw surfaces. Examples are dicophane dusting powder, zinc and salicylic acid dusting powder, zinc, starch and talc dusting powder.

DENTIFRICES

Dentifrices are substances or preparations which are generally used with the help of tooth brush for cleaning the surfaces of the teeth. They are available in the form of fine powders and pastes.

EAR DROPS

Ear drops are the liquid preparations in which the drug or drugs are dissolved or suspended in a suitable vehicle like water, dilute alcohol, glycerin or propylene glycol and are intended for instillation into the ear with a dropper. They are generally used for cleansing the ear, drying weeping surfaces, softening the wax and for treating the mild infections.

Ear drops are dispensed in coloured, fluted bottles attached with a dropper or in suitable plastic containers. The containers should be labelled "For external use only". Examples are hydrogen peroxide ear drops, phenol ear drops, etc.

ELIXIRS

Elixirs are clear, pleasantly flavoured, sweetened hydroalcoholic liquid preparations for oral administration. The main ingredients of elixirs are ethanol and water but glycerin, sorbitol, propylene glycol, flavouring agents, sugar and preservatives may be incorporated to the preparation. The elixirs may be medicated or non-medicated. The medicated elixirs usually contain very potent drugs such as antibiotics, antihistaminics and sedatives. The non-medicated elixirs are used as flavours and vehicles. Examples are chlorpheniramine elixir, diphenhydramine elixir, ephedrine elixir, paracetamol elixir, paediatric; piperazine citrate elixir, etc.

EMULSIONS

Emulsions are the biphasic liquid dosage form of medicament in which two immiscible liquids (generally one of which is water and the other is some lipid or oil) are made miscible by the addition of a third substance known as emulgent or emulsifying agent. Emulsions are comparatively pleasant to take than to take an oil as such.

Emulsions are of two types (a) oil in water type (O/W) (b) water in oil type (W/O). The former is generally for oral administration whereas the latter is generally for application to the skin.

Emulsions should be supplied in wide mouthed containers labelled with "Shake the bottle before use" label. Examples of emulsion are castor oil emulsion, liquid paraffin emulsion, liquid paraffin and phenolphthalein emulsion, etc.

ENEMAS

Enemas are aqueous or oily solutions or suspensions intended for introduction into the rectum for their purgative, sedative, anthelmintic, anti-inflammatory or nutritive effects. They may also be used for X-ray examination of the lower bowel. Among the commonly used drugs in solution form which act as cleansing enemas include isotonic solution of sodium chloride, sodium bicarbonate 2%, sodium phosphate, magnesium sulphate, soap and a combination of these substances. The other drugs in the form of enemas include olive oil, arachis oil, chloralhydrate, paraldehyde, turpentine, alum, tannic acid, barium sulphate, etc.

Usually solutions in volume of 500 ml to 1000 ml, depending on the age and condition of the patient, are introduced as enema. However, the commercially available concentrated enemas are introduced in small volumes of 100 to 200 ml. Large volume enemas should be warmed to body temperature before administration. Examples are paraldehyde enema, soap enema, etc.

EYE DROPS

Eye drops are sterile aqueous or oily solutions or suspensions for instillation into the eye. They are usually applied into the space between the eyeball and eyelids or onto the corneal surface. The main requirement of eye drops is that they should be sterile, usually isotonic, buffered and free from foreign particles to avoid irritation to the eye. They usually contain substances having antiseptic, anaesthetic, anti-inflammatory, mydriatic or miotic properties or substances used for diagnostic purposes.

Eye drops should be dispensed in glass or suitable plastic containers with a screw cap fitted with a rubber teat and glass dropper for easy application of the drops or the containers may be fitted with a narrow nozzle from which the drops can be directly instilled into the eye. Examples are atropine eye drops, chloramphenicol eye drops, cocaine eye drops, hydrocortisone eye drops, hyoscine eye drops, pilocarpine eye drops, sulphacetamide eye drops, etc.

EYE LOTIONS

Eye lotions or eye washes are sterile aqueous solutions used for irrigating the eye. They are usually applied with a clean eye bath or sterile fabric dressing and a large volume of solution is allowed to flow quickly over the eye.

Eye lotions are usually supplied in concentrated form and are required to be diluted with an equal volume of warm water immediately before use. They should be freshly prepared and should not be stored for more than 2-3 days as they may be contaminated with microorganisms on prolonged storage. Eye lotions should be isotonic and free from foreign particles to avoid irritation to the eye. The drugs used for preparing eye solutions include sodium chloride, sodium bicarbonate, boric acid, borax and zinc sulphate.

Eye lotions should be dispensed in coloured fluted bottles. The container should be labelled "For external use only". Examples are sodium bicarbonate eye lotion and sodium chloride eye lotion.

GARGLES

Gargles are aqueous solutions used for the prevention or treatment of throat infections. Usually they are concentrated solutions and should be diluted with warm water before use. In using the gargles they are brought into intimate contact with the mucous membrane of the throat and are allowed to remain there for a few moments after which they are thrown out of the mouth. Some of the analgesic preparations like aspirin gargles may be swallowed afterwards.

Gargles should be dispensed in white fluted bottles.

GELS

Generally gels are the aqueous colloidal suspensions of the hydrated forms of insoluble inorganic drugs. Examples are aluminium hydroxide gel, aluminium phosphate gel, milk of magnesia, etc. They are generally used as antacid.

GLYCERINS

They are also known as glycerites. Glycerins are the viscous preparations in which the drug is dissolved in glycerin with or without heating. They are generally used as antiseptic or anti-inflammatory preparations. Examples are ichthammol glycerin, phenol glycerin, tannic acid glycerin, etc.

GRANULES

Granules are the solid dosage form of medicament in which the powdered drug or drugs are mixed with sweetening, flavouring and colouring agents. A suitable granulating agent is added to moisten the powder and mixed thoroughly. The wet mass is passed through a suitable sieve and granules dried at a temperature of 60°C. They are supplied in glass containers and the patient is asked to add sufficient freshly boiled and cooled water to constitute a liquid preparation.

EFFERVESCENT GRANULES

These are specially prepared solid dosage form of medicament, meant for internal use. They usually contain citric acid, tartaric acid, sodium bicarbonate and medicament. A sweetening agent such as saccharin or sucrose may be incorporated.

When these granules are added to water, the acids react with sodium bicarbonate to liberate carbon dioxide and the preparation is taken while effervescing or immediately afterwards. These preparations act as antacid.

IMPLANTS

Implants are sterile small tablets meant for insertion under the skin by giving a small cut into the skin which is stitched afterwards. They are used to provide slow and continuous release of the drug for a long time ranging from 3 to 6 months or even more. These tablets are more commonly used in animals than human beings. Generally steroidal hormones like testosterone, stilbesterol, etc. are formulated as implants.

INFUSIONS

Infusions are liquid preparations which are either prepared by infusion process or by diluting 1 part of concentrated infusion with 9 parts of water. Infusions should be freshly prepared and must be used within 12 hours of their preparation. Examples are concentrated compound gentian infusion and concentrated senega infusion.

INHALATIONS

Inhalations are the liquid preparations containing volatile ingredients. They are used to relieve nasal congestion and inflammation of the respiratory tract. They may be placed on a pad or added to hot water and vapours inhaled for five to ten minutes. Examples are benzoin inhalation, menthol and eucalyptus inhalation.

INJECTIONS

Injections are the sterile liquid preparations containing one or more medicaments dissolved or suspended in a suitable vehicle and are meant for introduction into the body tissues by means of an injection under or through one or more layers of the skin or mucous membrane. Examples are ampicillin injection, dextrose intravenous infusion, gentamycin injection, etc.

INSUFFLATIONS

These are the finely divided powders meant for introduction into the body cavities such as ears, nose, tooth sockets and vagina with the help of an apparatus known as insufflator to which it would be difficult to apply the powder directly.

IRRIGATIONS

These are the solutions containing medicaments used to treat infections of the bladder, vagina and nose. These are introduced into the cavities by means a soft rubber tube known as catheter. They are generally used as antiseptic, anti-inflammatory or cleansing solutions.

JELLIES

Jellies are transparent or translucent non-greasy semisolid preparations meant for external application to the skin or mucous membrane. They are used for medication or lubrication purposes. Some of them are also used as contraceptive jellies. Examples are proflavin jelly, ichthammol jelly, etc.

LINCTUSES

Linctuses are sweet, viscous liquid preparations usually containing medicinal substances which have demulcent, sedative or expectorant properties. They are used for the treatment of cough. Linctuses are swallowed slowly in small doses without addition of water. Examples are codeine linctus, noscapine linctus, etc.

LINIMENTS

Liniments are liquid or semiliquid preparations meant for external application to the skin. Liniments are applied by rubbing or friction but should not be applied to the broken skin. They should be dispensed in coloured fluted bottles in order to distinguish from preparations meant for external use. The bottle should be labelled "For external use only" and "Shake the bottle before use". Examples are soap liniment, white liniment, etc.

LOTIONS

Lotions are liquid suspensions or dispersions meant for external application to the skin without friction. They usually contain alcohol and glycerin because alcohol hastens drying and produces cooling sensation whereas glycerin keeps the skin moist for a sufficient long time.

Lotions should be dispensed in a coloured fluted bottle with "For external use only" and "Shake the bottle before use" label. Examples are calamine lotion and salicylic acid lotion.

LOZENGES

Lozenges are the solid dosage form of medicament which are meant for slow dissolution in the mouth. Along with medicament they contain a sweetening agent, flavouring agent and a strong binding agent. They may be prepared either by moulding or by compression. Examples are compound bismuth lozenges, liquorice lozenges, etc.

MIXTURES

Mixtures are liquid dosage form of medicament in which drug or drugs are dissolved or suspended in a suitable aqueous vehicle. They may be sweetened and flavoured. They are freshly prepared and consumed within a few days. Mixtures are meant for oral administration and generally several doses are contained in a bottle. When only one dose is there, it is known as haustus or draught.

For indiffusible solids a suitable suspending agent will have to be incorporated to make the substance diffusible, so as to measure the dose easily. The containers of such mixtures should be labelled "Shake the bottle before use". Examples are aluminium hydroxide mixture, kaolin mixture, magnesium sulphate mixture, etc.

MOUTHWASHES

Mouthwashes are usually aqueous solutions in concentrated form with a pleasant taste and flavour used for rinsing, deodorant, refreshing or antiseptic action. Medicated mouthwashes may contain astringents, antibacterial agents, protein precipitants or other agents. They are generally used after dilution with warm water on the mucous membrane of the mouth. Examples are compound sodium chloride mouthwash and zinc sulphate and zinc chloride mouthwash.

NASAL DROPS

Nasal drops are usually aqueous solutions intended for instillation into the nostrils by means of a dropper. They are commonly used for their antiseptic, local analgesic or vasoconstrictor properties. Examples are ephedrine nasal drops.

OINTMENTS

Ointments are the soft semisolid preparations meant for external application to the skin or mucous membrane. They usually contain a medicament dissolved, suspended or emulsified in the base. Ointments are used for their emollient and protective action to the skin. Examples are compound benzoic acid ointment, calamine ointment, cetrimide emulsifying ointment, etc.

OPHTHALMIC OINTMENTS

Ophthalmic ointments are meant for application to the eye. They should be sterile and free from irritation. They should be packed in sterile containers which should keep the preparation sterile until whole of it is used up. Examples are atropine eye ointment, chloromycetin eye ointment.

PAINTS

Paints are the liquid preparations meant for external application to the skin or mucous membrane. They generally have a volatile solvent which evaporates quickly to leave a dry film of the medicament. Throat paints are viscous preparations which are applied to the throat. They contain high contents of glycerin due to which the preparations remain sticking to the site of application and prolong the action of the medicament. Examples are coal tar paint, compound iodine paint.

PASTES

Pastes are semisolid preparations meant for external application to the skin. They differ from ointments in that they generally contain a large amount of finely powdered solids such as starch, zinc oxide, calcium carbonate, etc. They provide a protective coating over the areas to which they are applied. They may be applied directly to the affected part or by spreading on a suitable backing material which is then applied to the affected area. Examples are magnesium sulphate paste, zinc and coal tar paste.

PESSARIES

Pessaries are the solid unit dosage form of medicament meant for introduction into the vagina. The bases used for the manufacture of pessaries are such that at room temperature they retain the original shape but when inserted into the cavity either melt or dissolve in the cavity fluids to release the medicament. They may be prepared either by moulding or by compression. Examples are lactic acid pessaries, nystatin pessaries.

POWDERS

Powders are solid dosage form of medicament meant for internal and external use. The powders meant for internal use are known as oral powders whereas those meant for external use are known as dusting powders. The powders may be simple or compound. When the powders are dispensed in large quantities in a container and the patient is asked to measure a specified quantity as a base then these powders are known as bulk powders. Examples are compound rhubarb oral powder, compound sodium chloride and dextrose oral powder, talc dusting powder, etc.

SOLUTIONS

Solutions are liquid preparations meant for internal or external use. They contain one or more than one ingredient usually dissolved in water. They may be sterile when intended for parenteral administration or unsterilized when intended for oral administration. Examples are strong ammonium acetate solution, aqueous iodine solution, cetrimide solution, etc.

SOLUTION TABLETS

Solution tablets contain a medicament or medicaments required to dissolve completely in the liquid to produce solutions of definite concentration. The solutions prepared by dissolving the soluble tablets may include mouthwashes, gargles, skin lotions, douches, antibiotics and certain vitamins. Examples are effervescing mouthwash tablets, benzyl penicillin solution tablets.

SPIRITS

Spirits are solutions of medicament or medicaments in alcohol (90 per cent). Examples are chloroform spirit, lemon spirit, compound orange spirit.

SPRAYS

Sprays are the liquid preparations of medicaments in aqueous, alcoholic or glycerin containing vehicle and are meant for application to the nose or throat by means of an atomiser or nebuliser. Examples are compound adrenaline and atropine spray, isoprenaline spray.

SUPPOSITORIES

Suppositories are special shaped solid dosage form of medicament for insertion into body cavities other than mouth. They may be inserted into rectum, vagina or urethra. These products are so formulated that after insertion they will either melt or dissolve in the cavity fluids to release the medicament. Suppositories vary in shapes, sizes and weights. Generally suppositories from 1 to 2 gm are prepared with either cocoa butter or glycerogelatin base. Examples are aminophylline suppositories, glycerol suppositories, etc.

SUSPENSIONS

Suspensions are the biphasic liquid dosage form of medicament in which the finely divided solid particles ranging from 0.5 to 5.0 micron are suspended or dispersed in a liquid or semisolid vehicle. Suspensions are mainly used for oral administration, external application or parenteral use. Examples are barium sulphate suspension, chalk, kaolin suspension.

SYRUPS

Syrups are sweet, viscous, concentrated aqueous solutions of sucrose or other sugars in water or any other suitable aqueous vehicle. They are used as sweetening and flavouring agents. Examples are lemon syrup, raspberry syrup, tolu syrup, etc.

TABLETS

Tablets are unit solid dosage form of medicament or medicaments with or without suitable diluents. They are prepared by moulding or usually by compression. Tablets are generally meant for oral administration but may be used by other routes of administration. Examples are aminophylline tablets, chloroquine sulphate tablets, paracetamol tablets, etc.

TINCTURES

Tinctures are alcoholic liquid preparations containing the active principles of vegetable drugs. They are usually prepared by maceration or percolation, or may be prepared by dissolving the corresponding liquid extract or chemical substances in alcohol or hydroalcoholic solvent. Examples are belladonna tincture, aromatic cardamom tincture, nux vomica tincture, etc.

THROAT PAINTS

Throat paints are viscous liquid preparations used for mouth and throat infections. Glycerin is commonly used as a base because of viscous nature and agreeable taste. Examples are boroglycerin, phenol glycerin and compound iodine paint (Mandl's paint).

Containers and Closures
(Packaging of Pharmaceuticals)

Packaging is the process by which the pharmaceuticals are suitably packed so that they should retain their therapeutic effectiveness from the time of their packaging till they are consumed. Packaging may be defined as the art and science which involves preparing the articles for transport, storage, display and use. An utmost care might have been taken during the formulation of any preparation but if it is not packaged properly the whole aim may be lost. Different shapes and sizes of containers made from different materials are used for packing different types of formulations. Therefore a careful consideration must be given for the selection of packaging material. A package may consist of:

1. **Container.** A container may be defined as a device in which the drug is enclosed and is in direct contact with the drug. A container which remains in contact with the drug at all times is known as immediate container.

2. **Closure.** A closure is a device which seals the container to exclude oxygen, carbon dioxide, moisture, microorganisms and prevent the loss of volatile substances. It also prevents the loss of medicament during transport and handling. A closure is considered as a part of container system. It does not come in direct contact with the medicament.

3. **Carton.** Carton is the outer covering which gives secondary protection against mechanical and other environmental hazards. They are made from cardboard, moulded wood pulp or expanded polystyrene.

4. **Box.** A box is a device which is generally used for packing multiples of the product. It gives primary protection against external hazards during transport and handling. A box is usually made from thick cardboard, wood or any other suitable material.

CHARACTERISTICS OF CONTAINERS AND CLOSURES

1. The container must be sufficiently strong to withstand handling while empty, when filling, closing, sterilizing, labelling, transport, storage and use by the consumer.
2. They should not allow any loss of product due to leakage, spillage or permeation.
3. The material of the container from which they are prepared must not react with the contents.
4. They must be able to withstand heat if process includes sterilization by heat.
5. The surface of the container must be clear for easy labelling.
6. The container must not absorb substances from the preparation e.g. absorption of water and oily substances from ointments and creams by the cardboard boxes.
7. The container must not impart its own colour, taste and odour to the preparation.
8. The container and closure must not react either with each other or with the preparation.
9. The container should be able to protect light-sensitive preparations for which amber-coloured glass containers may be used.
10. The size of the container must be selected according to the size of the preparation.
11. The closure must be easy to remove and replace.
12. The cost of container and closure is an integral part of overall cost of the preparation so it should not be high.
13. A container should facilitate the identification of a product i.e. whether meant for internal or external use.
14. Apart from all these characteristics a container and closure should be attractive in appearance and must have sale promotional and marketing values.

According to the method of closure and use, the containers are of following types:

1. Well-Closed Containers

A well-closed container is used to protect the preparation from contamination by extraneous solids, to prevent the loss of potency of active constituents and to prevent the loss of contents during transport, storage and handling.

2. Air-Tight Containers

Air-tight containers are used to protect the containers from atmospheric contamination of liquids, solids or vapours. They prevent the loss of drugs due to efflorescence, deliquescence or evaporation.

3. Hermetically-Sealed Containers

Hermetically-sealed container is that which does not allow the air and other gases to pass through it. Generally these types of containers are used for injectables. A glass ampoule sealed by fusion is the most common example of these types of containers.

4. Light-Resistant Containers

Light-resistant containers are used to protect the drugs which undergo decomposition in the presence of light. Such drugs may be enclosed in light-resistant amber-coloured or opaque containers.

5. Single Dose Containers

They are used to supply only one dose of the medicament. They are sealed in such a way that the contents cannot be removed without removing the seal. The contents so removed are consumed immediately e.g. ampoules.

6. Multi-Dose Containers

A multidose container holds a number of doses. It is sealed in such a way that successive doses can be withdrawn easily without changing the strength, quality or purity of the remaining contents e.g. multidose vials.

7. Aerosol Containers

Containers for aerosols must be strong enough to withstand the pressure evolved inside the container at the time of use of the preparation.

CLASSIFICATION OF CONTAINERS ACCORDING TO THEIR SHAPES

1. Glass/polythene bottles
   (i) Narrow mouth
   (ii) Wide mouth
2. Dropper bottles
3. Collapsible tubes
4. Gallipots
5. Cardboard boxes
6. Ampoules
7. Vials
8. Polythene packets for intravenous fluids
9. Polythene bottles for intravenous fluids
10. Aerosol containers
11. Envelops, strips, cartons, boxes, drums, etc.

Liquid oral preparations, intended to be swallowed like mixtures, emulsions, linctuses, syrups, oral gels, draughts etc., are required to be dispensed in narrow mouth bottles made from glass or polythene.

Liquid preparations, which are not to be swallowed like gargles, throat paints and mouthwashes, should be packed in fluted or ribbed bottles so that from its characteristic feel the patient may come to know that the preparation is not to be swallowed.

Liquid preparations like applications, liniments, lotions, paints, etc. meant for external application to the skin should generally be supplied in coloured fluted bottles in order to distinguish them from preparations meant for internal use.

Eye drops, ear drops, nasal drops, etc. should be dispensed in amber-coloured glass bottles fitted with a dropper. Now a days manufacturers prefer a plastic squeeze bottle with a plastic cap to which a dropper device is attached. This type of arrangement has the advantage that whole of the medicament is not exposed to atmospheric conditions. When in use, the entire medicament is not contaminated as a few drops are instilled into the cavity while the dropper is still in its position. The chances of spillage of liquid from the container are eliminated.

Semisolid preparations like ointments, creams, pastes etc. are dispensed in wide mouth containers or gallipots. On manufacturing scale collapsible tubes made from metal or plastic are preferred because:

(i) Their narrow opening prevents the contamination of rest of the contents because the material once removed from the tube cannot re-enter it.

(ii) Wastage is reduced because patient will remove only the required amount of medicament.

(iii) Nozzle type applicators may be attached to the tube to facilitate introduction into the body cavities such as nose, vagina or anus.

Individual powders are dispensed in paperboard or plastic boxes or paperboard cartons. Bulk powders and granules for internal use are usually packed in wide mouth, screw capped, colourless glass jars but plastic containers and paper lined aluminium containers may also be used.

Dusting powders and insufflations are dispensed in air-tight, wide mouthed, glass or plastic jars with instructions to the patient to use the powder with a swab of clean cotton wool or gauge. Proprietary dusting powders are packed in metal sifter-top containers.

Solid dosage forms like tablets, lozenges, hard and soft capsules are generally packed in strips made from cellophane or tin foil. For bulk packing either amber-coloured vials or bottles are used which are closed with plastic or metal screw caps that contain a suitable insert. Suppositories and pessaries prepared by compression may be packed similar to that of tablets or capsules but suppositories prepared by moulding are wrapped individually in waxed paper or tin foil which is then packed in shallow partitioned paperboard boxes. Now a days suppositories are prepared in a strip of disposable plastic moulds.

MATERIALS USED FOR THE CONSTRUCTION OF CONTAINERS

The following materials are used for the construction of containers. They are used either singly or sometimes in combination with each other.

1. Glass
2. Plastics
3. Metals
4. Paper.

1. Glass

Glass is mostly produced by heating a mixture of silica (SiO_2), soda ash (Na_2CO_3) and lime stone ($CaCO_3$) in a furnace at about 1400°C. The fused mass on rapid cooling forms glass which is soft in nature and is used for making bottles, light bulbs, etc. But if potassium carbonate is used instead of sodium carbonate, a hard glass is produced which is used for the preparation of laboratory glass apparatus. Special types of glass e.g. coloured glass or heat-resistant glass can be produced by adding certain other substances to the three basic components.

Various types of glass used for pharmaceutical purposes are:

(a) Type I — Borosilicate glass
(b) Type II — Treated soda-lime glass
(c) Type III — Soda-lime glass
(d) Type NP — Non-parenteral glass
(e) Coloured glass
(f) Neutral glass

(a) Type I — Borosilicate Glass

Borosilicate glass is produced by replacing the sodium oxide flux by boric oxide (B_2O_3) and some of lime by alumina (Al_2O_3) in the basic components of glass. It has a high melting point and can withstand high temperatures; hence it does not crack when used for boiling the water and even for cooking. It is also resistant to chemical substances. This type of glass is mainly used for making laboratory glass apparatus in factories, kitchens and ovens.

(b) Type II — Treated Soda Lime Glass

It is prepared from commercial soda-lime glass by treating it with sulphur dioxide by which surface alkali is de-alkanised and such glass can be used for alkali-sensitive products.

Sometimes inner surface of glass is treated with silicones and the glass so treated can be used for alkali sensitive products. Silicon treated glass is not very popular with pharmaceutical manufacturers due to flaking.

(c) Type III — Soda Lime Glass

It is an ordinary glass prepared from silicon dioxide soda ash (for Na_2O) and lime stone (for CaO) and is generally referred to as soda lime glass. It is the cheapest quality and most common form of glass. It contains a high concentration of alkaline oxides and imparts alkalinity to aqueous substances readily which can adversely effect the quality of the product contained therein. So these types of glasses are not suitable for alkali-sensitive products. They should not be used for parenteral preparations. These types of containers are generally used for solid medicaments.

(d) Type NP — Non-parenteral Glass

It is general purpose soda-lime glass used for oral and topical preparations.

(e) Coloured Glass

Coloured glass is obtained by adding small amounts of metal salts during fusion of glass. Coloured glass is used for light-sensitive products. For this purpose amber-coloured glass is generally used which does not allow the UV rays to pass through it. Preferably coloured glass should not be used for parenteral products because it becomes difficult to check clarity in such preparations.

(f) Neutral Glass

It is another commercial variety of glass available in between soda lime glass and borosilicate glass. It is resistant to alkalies, weathering and can withstand autoclaving. It is used for the manufacture of multidose vials and transfusion bottles, etc. It is composed of SiO_2 75%, B_2O_3 7-10%, Na_2O 6-8%, Al_2O_3 4-6%, BaO 2-4%, K_2O 0.5-2%.

For the manufacture of ampoules special glass tubing having low melting point should be used because after filling the ampoules are required to be sealed by fusion of glass.

Flaking

During flaking the alkali is extracted from the surface of glass containers and a silica rich layer is formed which sometimes gets detached from the surface and can be seen in the contents in the form of shining flakes. This is a serious problem specially in parenteral preparations. Therefore glass which does not flake should be selected.

Weathering

Weathering is a common problem with glass containers. Sometimes moisture condensed on the surface of glass container can extract some weakly bounded alkali, leaving behind a white deposit of alkali carbonate. If this white deposit is not removed and allowed to remain over there, further condensation of moisture will lead to the formation of an alkaline solution which will dissolve some silica resulting in loss of brilliance. This loss of brilliance from the surface of glass is called weathering. To prevent weathering, the deposited white layer of alkali carbonates should be removed as early as possible by washing the container with a dilute solution of acid and then washing thoroughly with water.

Sometimes glass free from lead and arsenic is used for those preparations which can extract lead or arsenic from the containers.

Due to flaking and weathering, all the glass apparatuses used for pharmaceutical purposes must be free from alkali and all the containers used therein must have passed the limit tests for alkalinity as prescribed in various pharmacopoeias.

Advantages of Glass Containers

1. They are transparent which allows the visual inspection of the contents.
2. They are economical.
3. They are readily available in various shapes and sizes.
4. They are chemically inert.
5. They are quite strong and rigid.
6. They possess superior protection properties.
7. They do not deteriorate with age, with proper closures.
8. Some glass containers are heat resistant so they can be readily sterilized by heat.
9. Glass containers can be easily cleaned without any damage to its surface e.g. scratching or bruising.
10. As the composition of glass may be varied by adding suitable amounts and types of sand and silica as well as conditions of heat treatment used, the proper container according to desired qualities can be produced.

Disadvantages

1. They are brittle and break easily.
2. They may crack when subjected to sudden changes of temperatures.
3. Some containers impart alkalinity and insoluble flakes to the formulations. This type of difficulty can be overcome by selecting proper type of glass.

2. Plastics

Plastics are high molecular weight polymers possessing long carbon chains. They are synthetic polymers which are converted into different forms. There are two types of plastics (i) thermosetting type, and (ii) thermoplastic type.

The thermosetting type plastics are usually hard and brittle at room temperature but become flexible on heating. They are used for making the closures for bottles and jars.

The thermoplastic type plastics are becoming more popular day be day. This type of plastic is used for the manufacture of plastic containers which are mainly used for packing mixtures, tablets, capsules, ointments, etc. I/V fluids and retention enemas are now packaged in plasticised PVC 'sachet' packs. These types of plastics have characteristic property that on heating they soften to become viscous fluids while on cooling again hardens. The various thermoplastic polymers used for the manufacture of containers are:

1. **Low density polythene.** It is used for the manufacture of bottles, jars, collapsible tubes, etc.

2. **High density polythene.** It is also used for bottles, jars and closures.

3. **Polyvinyl chloride (PVC).** It is of two types:

(a) Unplasticised which is used for bottles and jars.

(b) Plasticised which is used for making extruded tubes and films.

4. **Polystyrene.** It is used for jars, tubes and closures, etc. but is not suitable for the moisture sensitive products.

5. **Polypropylene.** It is used for the manufacture of squeeze bottles. It has a melting point of 170°C and containers made from it can be sterilized by autoclaving. It has a drawback that it becomes brittle at low temperatures.

6. **Polymethylmethacrylate (PMMA).** It is clear, hard, strong and light and is used for the manufacture of bottles, tubes, etc. It has the drawback that at low temperatures it becomes soft therefore not very suitable for containers of sterile products.

7. **Polytetrafluoroethylene (PTFE).** It has high resistance to heat and can withstand a temperature upto 250°C. It is also resistant to chemicals and its permeability to water vapours is also very low. It is very costly due to which it is not so commonly used in pharmaceutical practice.

8. Polyamides (Nylons). Nylons are very tough materials but at the same time they are also very flexible. They are resistant to heat with melting point of about 200°C. They are also resistant to chemicals. Nylons can be easily sterilized by autoclaving.

Sometimes in addition to above mentioned basic polymers, other additives such as plasticizers, antioxidants, colouring agents, etc. may be incorporated. Since these additives do not form bonds with the basic polymers so they may transmit to the preparation on storage, resulting to spoil the product.

Before packing the pharmaceutical products into the plastic containers they must be physically, chemically and biologically tested to ensure safety and stability of the preparation. The containers must be free from toxicity, irritability and pyrogens, etc., whenever necessary. Plastic containers meant for photosensitive materials should be tested for penetration of ultraviolet rays. Whenever coloured containers are used, it must be ensured that the colour is not transmitted to the preparation.

Advantages of Plastic Containers

1. They are cheaper as compared to other containers.
2. They can be readily produced on large scale.
3. They are unbreakable, tough and flexible.
4. They are light in weight and can be easily transported.
5. They can be moulded into various shapes and sizes.

3. Metals

Metal containers are not very popular for packing the pharmaceutical products because they may react with the preparations, have considerable weight and are costlier. Metal containers are, however, used for packing aerosols, powders, tablets and food articles. For this purpose tin-plated steel, stainless steel and aluminium containers are used.

Collapsible tubes made from aluminium, tin and lead are used but aluminium tubes are most popular because they are cheap as compared to tubes made from tin. Collapsible tubes are used for packing ointments, creams, pastes, tooth pastes and cosmetics. They are attractive containers and allow only the desired amount of the product to be removed. They do not allow the product to be contaminated as the rest of the preparation will not come in contact neither with the fingers not with the atmosphere. Collapsible tubes are light in weight, unbreakable and can be filled easily at a high speed with automatic machines.

Collapsible tubes are available in different sizes. Sometimes they are supplied with nozzles which can be attached to the tube for ease in application of the medicament to the nose, rectum or other body cavities.

4. Paper

Paper and board as packing material are widely used in pharmaceutical industries in one form or the other. They are used to prepare containers ranging from envelops used for dispensing powders, a few tablets or a few capsules on the counter, to the drums used for storing large quantities of drugs in the industries. Cartons and boxes made from board are used for packing the pharmaceutical containers.

Properties of paper and board can be modified by treating it with plastic, wax or other materials. Such treated paper will protect the products from atmospheric conditions. Now a days chemically treated paper known as tetrapack paper is also available for storing the drugs and chemicals.

MATERIALS USED FOR THE CONSTRUCTION OF CLOSURES

1. Cork
2. Glass
3. Plastics
4. Rubber
5. Metals

1. Cork

Cork is essentially a wood obtained from the bark of oak tree. It is used for the manufacture of stoppers for narrow mouth bottles. Cork is almost chemically inert and does not impart undesirable odour or flavour to the preparation. The main disadvantage of these closures is that sometimes they lead to mould growth when used for aqueous preparations and may shed particles to products if not used carefully.

2. Glass

As compared to cork, glass is an ideal material for making the stoppers but these stoppers have the difficulties that they do not provide leak-proof closures. Moreover they can slip out of neck of the containers easily during transport and handling. Therefore the use of glass closures is restricted to laboratory glass apparatus e.g. reagent bottles and fancy cut glass items only.

3. Plastics

As compared to cork, glass, rubber and metal closures, plastic closures are becoming more popular day by day because they are unbreakable, light in weight, can be easily moulded into various shapes and sizes. Plastic closures selected must be tested before use for any extractive material present in them and for their reaction with the product contained in the bottle.

4. Rubber

Natural rubber consists of latex obtained from Heavea braziliensis commonly known as rubber plant. This rubber imparts a characteristic odour to the product. Therefore the physical and chemical properties of rubber are altered by the addition of some additives such as:

(a) Vulcanising agent e.g. sulphur.
(b) Accelerators e.g. thiazoles.
(c) Activators e.g. zinc oxide, stearic acid and zinc stearate.
(d) Fillers e.g. carbon black, calcium carbonate, zinc oxide, talc, etc.
(e) Softners e.g. mineral oils, etc.
(f) Antioxidants.
(g) Pigments e.g. oxides and sulphides of iron, cadmium, etc.
(h) Lubricants e.g. zinc stearate, etc.

Rubber closures are mainly used for vials, multidose containers and I/V fluid bottles because of its self-sealing properties and it can withstand sterilization temperatures better than plastic closures. Rubber is also used for making the washers required in certain containers.

Since the additives used in the manufacture of rubber has the tendency to migrate into the product contained in the container therefore these closures must be subjected to extractive test before use. The other tests which should be performed on rubber closures include (i) test for penetrability force, (ii) fragmentation test, (iii) permeability test and compatibility with the product.

QUALITIES OF AN IDEAL RUBBER CLOSURE

1. It should provide air-tight closing to the container.
2. It should be compatible with the preparation contained in the container.

3. It should not migrate any additive to the preparation.
4. It should withstand the sterilization temperatures.
5. It should be soft and elastic in nature so as to allow the hypodermic needle to pass through it easily but as soon as the needle is removed it should again provide the perfect seal.

Synthetic rubbers are costly; so not very commonly used for the manufacture of closures.

Advantages of Rubber

1. Rubber does not deteriorate with age. Under normal conditions closures prepared from good quality rubber remain stable for a number of years.
2. Rubber acts as self-seal to the containers.
3. Rubber is elastic in nature and can be moulded in any form to make stoppers or closure liners. It is elastic enough that it provides a snug fit between the closure and the neck and lip of the glass container. They are soft and elastic enough that they allow easy passage to the syringe needle without blunting and springs back to its original position to close the hole made by the needle immediately after withdrawal to prevent the entry of microorganisms and leakage of the contents.
4. Although porous they do not allow the transfer of water vapours or gases in either direction.
5. Good quality rubber is resistant to sterilization conditions.
6. They are unbreakable, tough and can be easily transported.

Disadvantages of Rubber

1. The composition of rubber stoppers is complex and the manufacture process is complicated.
2. When rubber stopper comes in contact with parenteral solutions, it may absorb the active medicament, preservative or other materials, and one or more constituents of the rubber may be extracted into the liquid which may (a) interfere with the chemical analysis of the active medicament, (b) affect the toxicity or pyrogenicity of the parenteral preparation, (c) lose or decrease the preservation and physical stability of the preparation.
3. Hard rubber may produce large number of fragments when the hypodermic needle cuts through the closure and the fragmented material may appear in the solution.

5. Metals

Tin plate and aluminium are most commonly used for the manufacture of closures but aluminium is most widely used for this purpose because it is ductile in nature and closure of any desired shape and size can be easily manufactured with it. Further, tear off closures can only be made from aluminium. To make the closures pilfer-proof they may be sealed with aluminium cap in such a way that its central part is easily removed at the time of administration of the preparation but the cap itself should remain in position, if so desired.

CLOSURE LINERS

Closure liners are the materials which are placed in a closure to make it pilfer-proof and prevent the decomposition of the product due to moisture, bacterial or fungal growth. Almost all types of closures except glass stoppers must be packed with a suitable liner which may include cork, rubber, pulp board, plastic and felt.

Types of Closures

1. Once-only closures e.g. fusion of glass to seal an ampoule or fusion of plastic to seal a polyethylene bag.
2. Renewable closures — They are used for bottles, jars, tubes, etc. and is of following types:
    (a) Plug type e.g. closing the neck of the container with a cork or glass stopper but both of these have been replaced by plastic stoppers because they are unbreakable and flexible to ensure better fitting.
    (b) Cap type
       (i) Push fit caps e.g. closing of the tablet or capsule vials where the neck of the container and plastic cap is shaped in such a way that the cap fits well in the neck of the container and cap is stretched over it so as to provide a perfect seal.
       (ii) Screw closures — They are the most widely used closures for all types of containers having screwed neck but care must be taken that the cap should also be screwed to the correct extent.

STRIP OR BLISTER PACKAGING

Unit dosage form of drugs like tablets and capsules are enclosed individually in strip or blister packs. In strip packing the unit drugs are hermetically sealed in between strips of aluminium foil and/or plastic film. The contents are removed by tearing or cutting the individual pocket.

In blister packing the unit dosage forms are enclosed in between transparent blisters and suitable packing material, generally aluminium foil. The contents are removed simply by pushing the drug through the backing strip.

AEROSOLS

A pharmaceutical aerosol may be defined as the preparation containing the active medicament dissolved, suspended or emulsified in a propellant or a mixture of solvent and propellant and packaged in a pressurised aerosol container. When little pressure is applied on the valve attached to the pressurised container, the medicament is released in the form of a mist or an aerosol spray. For aerosol systems the propellants used include compressed gases such as carbon dioxide or nitrogen or liquefied gases like methane, ethane, etc. Liquefied gases are more commonly used as propellants because they maintain a constant pressure until last drop of the product is taken out of the container. For potent drugs used in asthma the valve includes a metering device which delivers only a metered dose on applying pressure on the valve. The patients should be warned not to exceed the prescribed dose.

Uses

Pressurised aerosols are becoming more popular day by day. They are used only in pharmaceutical practice but a large number of consumer items like cosmetics, perfumes, etc. are being packed in pressure aerosol containers in spite of high packing costs. Pharmaceutical pressurised aerosols are used as local applications, local anaesthetics, local analgesics, antiseptics, germicides, antibiotics, anti-inflammatory agents, local application to the ear, nose, throat, lungs, etc.

Advantages of Aerosols

1. The products are easy and convenient to apply and can be administered without the help of a nurse or a doctor as is required in the case of injections.
2. The onset of action is faster because the medicament is directly administered to the affected part.
3. The dispersion of medicament is very efficient.

4. There is no manual contact with the medicament and the affected parts.
5. The possibility of drug decomposition in GIT on oral administration is eliminated since no drug is to pass through GIT.
6. There is no contamination of the product from external sources.
7. The sterility of the sterile products is maintained since no microorganism can enter even when the valve is opened.
8. Controlled and uniform dose is released by the metered valves.
9. Hydrolysis of medicament can be prevented since propellants do not contain any water.
10. Oxidation is prevented as no air is present in the container.
11. The aerosol containers except clear glass containers protect the photosensitive medicaments.
12. A fine mist of the drug is produced for inhalation purposes.

Disadvantages of Aerosols

1. They are costlier.
2. The disposal of empty containers may be difficult because the remaining amount of propellant present in the exhausted containers continues to exert pressure.
3. Aerosol packs must not be exposed to higher temperatures because it may develop high pressure inside the container.
4. When the drug is not soluble in the propellant it may create difficulties in the formulation of aerosols.
5. Propellants may cause toxic reactions if inhalation therapy is continued for a long period of time.

FORMULATION OF PHARMACEUTICAL AEROSOLS

A pharmaceutical aerosol consists of following essential components:
1. Active medicament
2. Solvent
3. Propellant

The active medicament(s) is dissolved in a suitable solvent to which other ingredients such as stabilizers, antioxidants, preservatives, solubilizers or dispersing agents may be incorporated. To this a propellant or a blend of propellants is added to develop pressure inside the container and to expel the product from the container when the valve is opened. Propellants can be mixed with active medicaments in a number of ways, producing products with different characteristics. Various gases used as aerosol propellants include:

(i) Compressed gases like carbon dioxide, nitrogen and nitrous oxide. Out of these only nitrogen is more useful in aerosols because it is inert.

(ii) Liquefied gases include fluorinated and fluorochlorinated hydrocarbons. Although a large number of compounds are available but dichlorodifluoromethane, trichloromonofluoromethane and dichlorotetrafluoroethane are widely used propellants in most pharmaceutical aerosols.

AEROSOL CONTAINERS

An aerosol container assembly consists of following parts:

1. Container
2. Valve

1. *Container.* The container used for packaging the pharmaceutical aerosols must possess at least the following qualities that (a) it should be capable of maintaining the required high pressure (b) the material from which it is manufactured must be compatible with the contents. The aerosol containers are generally made from tin plate, aluminium, glass, plastic-coated glass and plastics. In addition to all these materials, stainless steel is used in special cases to prevent attack by the contents.

2. *Valve.* The valve mechanism is the most important part of an aerosol assembly. Its main function is to regulate the flow of the product from the container and to control the type of spray. The valve includes not only the basic valve mechanism but it includes the closure in which it is mounted, the gasket, the dip tube and the actuator.

Various types of valves are used in aerosols which include (a) continuous spray valves and (b) metering valves. In continuous spray valves the medicament is continuously released from the container unless the pressure is released from the actuator. Such valves include spray valves used for spray aerosols e.g. room deodorants, anaesthetics, disinfectants, etc.; foam valves used for foam producing aerosols e.g. shaving creams, vaginal contraceptive foam aerosols, etc., stream valves used for solid stream aerosols, e.g. tooth pastes, ointments, creams, etc.

Metered valves are used for potent drugs where a measured quantity of drug is required to be administered during each single operation of

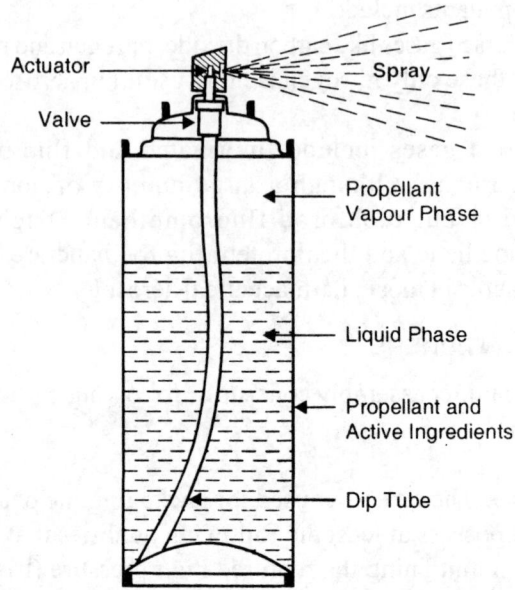

the actuator. These type of valves minimize the wastage and errors of overdosing of drugs.

An actuator is an integral part of each aerosol container which allows easy opening and closing of the valve. It is a specially designed button fitted to the valve stem which when pressed allows the contents to be released from the container in the form of an aerosol. There are different types of actuators available which may be used to produce spray, fine mist, foam or solid streams.

9

Sources of Errors and Care Required in Dispensing Prescriptions

WEIGHING METHODS

Weighing of substances is done in almost all types of pharmaceutical operations and is the first step in any compounding. The success of all these operations in pharmacy depends on a thorough knowledge of principles of the balance, its proper care and use.

Weighing generally refers to a definite weight of material to be used in compounding a prescription or manufacturing a dosage form. A balance may be defined as an instrument used to determine the relative weights of substances. Because balance is an important instrument for a pharmacist therefore it must be correctly selected, carefully used and properly checked after specified intervals of time to obtain accurate results. For prescription work generally dispensing balances are used which consist of a simple, light but rigid, equal armed, horizontal beam with central and terminal knife edges of steel which work in agate or steel bearing. Two pans are suspended from the terminal knife edges. When the load is placed in the pans the beam turns about the central fulcrum and deflection from the horizontal is indicated by movement of a pointer fixed below the centre of the beam. For weighing the materials the following techniques should be followed:

1. Place the balance in a well lighted location and in a convenient position for use. The area should be free from dust and there should be no corrosive vapours present nor high humidity or vibrations due to air currents.
2. Adjust the level of the balance.
3. Clean the pans with a clean cloth.
4. Place equal size powder papers (preferably wax paper) on each pan of the balance. They will prevent inaccuracy due to powder adhering to the pan and also to protect the pans from corrosion.
5. Place the required weights on the right hand pan with the help of forceps. The use of forceps will prevent inaccuracies in weighing due to sweat and grease from hands. Some of the writers suggest that the weights should be placed in the left hand pan and material to be weighed in the right hand pan. The left hand pan is less convenient because the pillar of the balance comes in the way but most of the workers prefer to use right hand pan for keeping the weights and left hand pan for keeping the material to be weighed.
6. Close the drawer of the balance which will prevent spillage of the powder on the weights lying in the drawer.
7. Remove the bottle of medicament from the shelf and check its label for the correct ingredient mentioned in the prescription.
8. Place the material to be weighed in the left hand pan. While taking out the material from the bottle hold the bottle in the left hand with the label upper most so that it is visible during weighing. Gently release the pan arrest to determine whether too much or too little material was added.
9. Remove or add the material, always using a spatula, after arresting the pan each time whenever transfer of material is made.
10. When the weights on the two pans will be equal the release of the pan arrest will show a zero rest point and the weighing is complete.
11. When the weighing is complete put the balance beam again in the fixed position.
12. Transfer the weighed material from the weighing paper to the compounding device and discard the weighing paper. Each time a new weighing paper should be used and readjusting of the balance equilibrium to a zero rest point must be done.
13. Return the weights to the drawer with forceps and carefully clean the balance pans and spatula.

14. Close the stock bottles and again check its labels. Return the bottles to the shelf. Preferably only one bottle should be removed from the shelf at a time for weighing and the same should be replaced immediately after the material is weighed. Then the next bottle should be removed and material weighed. This will avoid the mistakes which may be made if several bottles are kept on the bench together.

Possible Errors in Weighing

Errors in weighing may occur due to one or more of the following reasons:

1. If the balance is not leveled.
2. If the rest point of the balance is not correct.
3. If the two pans of the balance are of unequal weight.
4. If the pans are rough.
5. If the material is weighed directly on the pans.
6. If the weight of the material is taken while the pans are still oscillating.
7. If the weights are removed with fingers and not with forceps.
8. If the volatile substances are weighed in an open vessel.

Minimum Weighable Amounts

The maximum allowable error in weighing on a prescription balance is not more than ±5%. This value is significant only in very small weighings and efforts should be made to get a higher degree of accuracy. This figure indicates that of 100 mg of any substance is to be supplied then it must not be less than 95 mg and not more than 105 mg. But efforts should be made to weigh as near to 100 mg as possible. Since Smith's results showed that only 2 gr or more weighings were within ±5% errors therefore it is advisable not to weigh less than 100 mg (or 2 gr) on a prescription balance otherwise accurate weights will not be obtained. In any case amounts less than 50 mg (1 gr) should not be weighed on dispensing balance specially reserved for weighing quantities less than 100 mg or on general chemical balances.

Procedure for weighing below the minimum weighable amounts, geometrical dilutions

The practice of dispensing powders in very small doses is obsolete but still some practitioners write prescriptions of powders in very small doses. Therefore following procedures should be followed for dispensing quantities below the minimum weighable amounts:

1. Very small quantities of materials may be weighed on a high grade analytical balance but the cost of such a balance might be prohibitive because the number of prescriptions requiring its use may be few. Therefore this method is not commonly used.
2. Prefabricated dosage forms such as tablet triturates, dispensing tablets and hypodermic tablets of the same drug may be used. Though this method is very convenient but may introduce an error.
3. The use of liquid and solid dilutions is the most suitable and convenient means of dispensing the small amounts of drugs accurately. In this method a minimum weighable quantity of the drug is weighed on a dispensing balance which is then mixed with a solid diluent such as lactose (for solid dosage forms) or water or any other solvent (for liquid dosage forms). Lactose is selected as diluent because it is white, sweet in taste, easily available, cheap and compatible with majority of the drugs.

While preparing triturations and dilutions the following limiting factors must be kept in mind:

1. The quantity of active medicament to be diluted must not be less than the minimum weighable amount.
2. The final dilutions prepared must represent the desired amount of the drug in the minimum weighable amounts.

When a very small quantity of drug is to be dispensed the best method is to prepare triturations and dilutions by using lactose as diluent. The general procedure is as follows:

Weigh 100 mg (minimum weighable amount) of the drug. Mix it gradually or by means of geometrical dilutions with the required quantity of lactose. Then weigh a portion of the mixed material which will contain the desired weight of the potent drug.

TRITURATIONS

The term trituration is applied to a mixture or dilution of a potent substance with an inert substance. Small quantities of finely powdered solids may be mixed on a sheet of white paper by means of bone spatula or powder knife. If the quantities are large to be conveniently mixed on paper sheet then pestle and mortar should be used. The invariable rule is to add a small amount of the substance present in greater amount to whole of the substance present in lesser amount (generally potent substance) and mix thoroughly. The remaining amount of the substance present in larger amount is then incorporated gradually in small quantities at first which are subsequently increased until whole of it has been added. This method of mixing is known as geometrical dilutions which may be explained that when 100 mg of any potent drug is to be mixed with 900 mg of lactose the best method is to take out 100 mg of lactose from bulk and mix it with 100 mg of drug. Total of this mixture will be 100 + 100 = 200 mg. Again take out 200 mg of lactose and mix it with 200 mg of first mixture, total of this mixture will be 200 + 200 = 400 mg. In the next step again take out 400 mg of lactose and mix it intimately with the second mixed material, total of this will be 400 + 400 = 800 mg. To this 800 mg add whole of the remaining lactose and mix thoroughly so as to get a uniform powder.

By geometrical dilution method very small quantities of drugs can be mixed intimately with large quantities of diluents and a uniform powder will be obtained whereas it is impossible to get intimate dispersion of one powder in another by mixing the two substances all at once.

In the case of costly drugs it becomes necessary to give a thought to cost factor of the drug but under no circumstances the compounding accuracy should be compromised with economy.

Proper care and usage of dispensing balance

It is the general tendency of the pharmacists that they do not take proper care of balance while using it, cleaning it or protecting it while it is not used. As balance is the most important instrument for a pharmacist and in almost all kinds of prescriptions the need arises to use a balance at one stage or the other therefore proper care of a balance must be taken while using, cleaning and storing it. In this regard following points must be taken care of:

1. It should be kept in a place where there is no dust, dampness, corrosive vapours and vibrations.
2. The balance should be kept on a leveled surface which should be hard like bench or table.
3. The analytical balances are protected by enclosing in glass cases provided with doors in the front and in the sides. While weighing any substance these doors must be kept closed.

4. Always clean the pans and surfaces of the balance with a clean dry duster before its use as well as after its use.
5. While using a balance neither the weights nor the substance that is to be weighed should be kept on the pans while the beam is free to oscillate.
6. Greasy and waxy substances should be weighed on a carefully counterbalanced sheet of wax paper. Preferably all substances should be weighed by placing counterbalanced wax paper in each of the pans.
7. Substances which act as metals such as iodine, corrosive sublimate, etc., should not be weighed directly on the pans but on counterbalanced watch glass.
8. Any agent spilled on the balance during use should be wiped off immediately with a soft brush or cloth.
9. While weighing, the drawer of the balance should be closed.
10. Weights should be transferred with forceps.
11. All materials should be transferred with spatula.
12. While cleaning the balance great care should be taken so that the delicate mechanism of the balance is not disturbed. Soft cloth or brush should be used for cleaning the balance.
13. When the balance is not in use, it must be cleaned and covered with the balance cover.

If due consideration is given to the above mentioned points in handling and using the balance it may give accurate weighings, correct results and last for a long time.

10

Principles Involved and Procedures Adopted
in Dispensing of Typical Prescriptions

POWDERS

Powders are the solid dosage form of medicament which are meant for internal and external use. They are available in crystalline or amorphous form. Though the drugs are prepared in many different physical forms and shapes but many of them are prepared by using powders in one way or the other. Each dosage form so prepared has certain advantages over the other form. Similarly, the powders have certain advantages as described below:

1. Most of the drugs are available in powder forms and it becomes more convenient for the physician to prescribe specific amount of medicament according to the need of the patient.
2. Powders are usually more stable than liquids because chemical reactions take place more rapidly in atmospheric conditions when the drug is in liquid dosage form than powder.
3. Incompatibility is less in case of powders than liquids.
4. The smaller particle size of powders produces more rapid dissolution in the body fluids than other solid dosage forms of medicament, e.g., tablets, capsules or pills. The rapid dissolution increases the blood concentration in a shorter time, thereby the action is produced in a lesser time.

5. Large quantities of bulky drugs which are otherwise difficult to administer can be easily administered by mixing with liquids.
6. They are more easy to carry than liquids.
7. They are more economical as compared to other dosage forms because for extemporaneous preparation they do not require any special technique or machinery.
8. Children and old persons who cannot swallow solid dosage forms can easily injest powders which can be dispersed in water or any other liquid and may be administered through feeding tube to the patients who are fed by tubes which terminate in the stomach itself.

Disadvantages

1. Drugs which deteriorate on exposure to atmospheric conditions are not suitable for dispensing in powder forms.
2. Bitter, nauseous, corrosive and unpalatable drugs cannot be dispensed in powder form.
3. Deliquescent and hygroscopic drugs cannot be dispensed in powder form.
4. Volatile drugs are not suitable for dispensing in powder form.

CLASSIFICATION OF POWDERS

1. Simple and compound powders for internal use (Divided Powders).
2. Granular effervescent powders for internal use.
3. Bulk powders for external use, e.g., dusting powders, insufflations and tooth powders, etc.
4. Powders enclosed in catchets and capsules.
5. Compressed powders (Tablets) and tablet triturates.

Simple and Compound Powders

Simple Powders

A simple powder contains only one ingredient either in crystalline or amorphous form. When the powder is in the crystalline form, preferably it is reduced to fine powder, weighed and wrapped as individual doses as described in compound powders.

Rx

Aspirin   300 mg
Fiat pulvis. Mitte tales quarta.

Rx

Calcium gluconate   1 gm
Make powder. Send such six.

Compound Powders

Compound powders contain two or more than two substances which are mixed together and then divided into individual doses.

Rx

Aspirin	300 mg
Paracetamol	150 mg
Caffeine	50 mg

Fiat pulvis. Mitte tales octo.
Sig: Unus dolore urgente sumenda.
Type: Oral divided powder.

General Method of Preparation

Since there is little unavoidable loss of powder during weighing and mixing because some powder will adhere to the spatula, pestle and the mortar therefore calculate for one extra powder than required, but if by calculating for one extra powder an awkward fraction of weights is involved then a suitable number of extra powders may be calculated.

The dispensing balances are not so sensitive that the quantities less than 2 grain or 130 mg can be weighed accurately therefore the quantities weighing less than 2 grain or 130 mg must be triturated with a suitable inert diluent so that the quantities are made weighable on dispensing balance. Generally lactose is used as a diluent because it is colourless, soluble and compatible with majority of drugs. It is preferred to sucrose because sucrose has tendency to absorb moisture and become a cake.

Separately powder a slight excess of each crystalline substance. Weight out the required amount of each powder and diluent, i.e., lactose, if necessary. Mix all the ingredients in the ascending order of their weights and mix thoroughly so that a homogenous powder is formed.

Weigh out the required number of powders and wrap in the papers.

The volatile substances and hygroscopic powders require to be double wrapped, the inner wrapper of which should be of wax paper to prevent volatilization and absorption of moisture.

Marketed Powders

1. Acidin with belladonna powder (East India Pharmaceutical Works, Calcutta - 700071).
2. Bismag powder (Geoffrey Manners & Co. Ltd., Bombay - 400038).
   Contains:
   Sod. bicarbonate, heavy magnesium carbonate, light magnesium carbonate, calcium carbonate.
3. Prequest powder (sachet) [Parke-Davis (India) Ltd., Bombay - 400025].
   Contains:

Sod. chloride	0.365%
Sod. acid phos.	0.975%
Sod. citrate	1.839%
Pot. chloride	2.330%
Mag. sulphate	0.736%
Cal. lactate	0.545%
Dextrose anhydrous	89.900%

4. Raylyte powder (Rays Laboratories Pvt. Ltd., Calcutta - 700007).
   Each 27.5 gm contains:

Sod. chloride	3.5 gm
Sod. bicarbonate	2.5 gm
Pot. chloride	1.5 gm
Dextrose	20.0 gm

5. Takazyme powder [Parke-Davis (India) Ltd., Bombay - 400025].
   Each contains:

Mag. carbonate light	16%
Mag. trisilicate	8%

   Aspergillus (oryzae enzyme equ. to 1.07% alpha amylase)

POWDERS REQUIRING SPECIAL CONSIDERATIONS

1. Hygroscopic and Deliquescent Powders

Substances which absorb moisture from the atmosphere are not suitable for dispensing in powder papers because the absorbed moisture may promote the chemical degradation of the drug and in the case of effervescent preparations the acids may completely react with sodium bicarbonate rendering the preparation unfit for use. Among the commonly prescribed hygroscopic and deliquescent substances are ammonium chloride, ammonium bromide, ammonium iodide, calcium chloride, hyoscine hydrobromide, iron and ammonium citrate, pepsin, phenobarbitone sodium, potassium citrate, sodium bromide, sodium iodide, citric and tartaric acid.

When dispensing such powders, there are several precautions which a pharmacist must take to minimise absorption of moisture from the atmosphere. In first place the hygroscopic substances are usually supplied in granular form in order to expose less surface area to the atmosphere. These powders should not be finely powdered. If the need arises then the powdering may be carried out in a mortar which has been dried and warmed. Such powders should be double wrapped. In humid weather or when dealing with very deliquescent substances further wrapping in aluminium foil or plastic cover is advisable.

2. Eutectic Mixtures

When two or more substances are mixed together they liquefy due to the formation of a new compound which has a lower melting point than room temperature. The degree of liquefaction of eutectic substances is governed by their melting points, relative proportions and room temperature. The formation of eutectic mixtures signifies a physical change rather than a chemical change. The substances which on mixing liquefy are: menthol, acetanilide, thymol, phenacetin, camphor, aspirin, phenol, antipyrine, salol, chloral hydrate.

In dealing with eutectic substances firstly they may be dispensed as separate set of powders with directions that one set of each kind shall be taken as a dose. Secondly they may be incorporated in powders by adding an inert absorbent like magnesium carbonate, light magnesium oxide, kaolin, starch, lactose, calcium phosphate, bentonite, etc. Generally an equal amount of absorbent as that of eutectic substance is sufficient to prevent liquefaction. In this method each eutectic substance is mixed with an absorbent separately and then blended together lightly with a spatula on a sheet of paper. On the other hand when the substances which liquefy are present in small amount they may be mixed together so as to form a eutectic mixture, then the liquid so formed is absorbed by adding an absorbent. The remaining ingredients of the prescription are then incorporated and mixed together.

Rx

Menthol	5 gm
Camphor	5 gm
Ammonium chloride	30 gm
Light magnesium carbonate	60 gm

Fiat insufflatio. Mitte 50 gm.

Sig: Pro naso.

Type: Compound powder containing liquefiable substances.

3. Efflorescent Powders

Crystalline substances liberate water of crystallization wholly or partly due to change in relative humidity or during trituration, causing the powder to become wet or to liquefy. This difficulty may be overcome by using either corresponding anhydrous salt or an inert substance may be mixed with efflorescent substance before incorporating the other ingredients.

4. Vegetable Powders

Vegetable powders which contain volatile oils should not be subjected to heavy grinding in a mortar. When it is necessary to powder them, they must be powdered lightly in a mortar to prevent the loss of volatile oils present in them. In dispensing such vegetable powders and other volatile substances they must be double wrapped, inner wrapper of which should be of wax paper.

5. Liquids

If the quantity of the liquid to be incorporated is small, it may be triturated with an equal amount of powder, then the rest of the ingredients are incorporated in small portions with continuous trituration. If the quantities of liquids are large then an absorbent must be added.

Tinctures and fluid extracts will have to be evaporated but they should not be evaporated directly to dryness or a hard resinous mass which may be difficult to remove from the dish as well as difficult to mix with other ingredients. Therefore they must be partially evaporated until the liquid attains a syrupy consistency. Add lactose or any other suitable diluent and continue evaporation to dryness. Then incorporate other ingredients. The diluent is added to prevent the formation of sticky mass on evaporation. Whenever possible it is preferable to use powdered extracts instead of tinctures and fluid extracts in prescriptions.

6. Explosive Substances

When an oxidising agent and reducing agent are triturated in a mortar there are chances of explosion which may lead to serious consequences. Though the prescriptions for such combinations in powder form are rare, preferably should not be filled but if it has to be dispensed then powder each ingredient separately in a mortar and mix them lightly with other ingredients. Alternatively powder each substance separately and dispense them in separate powder paper with suitable directions to the patient regarding its use.

List of Oxidising and Reducing Agents

Oxidising agents	Reducing agents
Potassium chlorate	Charcoal
Potassium dichromate	Sulphur
Potassium nitrate	Sulphides
Potassium permanganate	Tannic acid
Silver nitrate	

Rx

Potassium chlorate	600 mg
Tannic acid	300 mg
Sucrose	300 mg

Fiat charta. Mitte tales tres.
Signa: Unus aqua cyathus gargarisma.

7. Potent Drugs

Substances having a maximum dose of less than one grain and poisonous substances should be regarded as potent substances. Small quantities of potent drugs should not be weighed on dispensing balance. The best method is to prepare triturations. These are dilutions of potent powdered drugs, prepared by intimate mixing of the drug with suitable diluent in definite proportion. In this method the drug is reduced to fine powder and to this an equal amount of diluent is mixed well by thorough trituration in a mortar. To this is incorporated the rest of the diluent in successive portions with thorough trituration each time until whole of the diluent has been added. Under no circumstances the whole of the diluent should be added to the drug at one time otherwise the potent drug will not be mixed uniformly and thoroughly in the diluent resulting in uneven dose in divided powders.

Rx

Prednisone   8 mg
Send such four powders.
Signa: One to be taken as directed.
Type: Simple divided potent powder.

Rx

Phenobarbitone sodium   15 mg
Send such 4 powders.
Sig: Unus omni nocte sumenda.
Type: Simple oral divided potent powder.

8. Granular Powders

Sometimes it is difficult to present solid medicaments with large doses in suitable dosage form. The tablets and capsules cannot be prescribed because a large number of them will be required to take as a single dose which is not feasible, liquids cannot be prepared because of stability problems. Therefore the choice remains to powders. But the bitter, nauseous and unpleasant powders are difficult to dispense as such, therefore these powders are prepared in the form of granules.

On a small scale the medicaments are mixed with sweetening, flavouring and colouring agents in a mortar. A suitable granulating agent is added to moisten the powders until the mass becomes coherent but not too damp. The granulating agents used may be water, starch mucilage, gelatin or sugar solutions and various dilutions of alcohol. Press down the coherent mass through sieve number 10 superimposed on sieve number 20 or 24. Dry the granules by spreading in a warm place for 2-3 hours or by keeping them in an oven at a temperature not exceeding 60°C. Pack them in dry, well closed, wide mouthed bottles.

On a large scale manufacturing various types of granulators are used for preparing the granules.

Now a days some of the antibiotics like erythromycin, nystatin, phenoxymethyl penicillin, etc., which are unstable in solution are prepared in the dry granular form in which the drug is mixed with suspending, sweetening, flavouring, colouring and granulating agents. The granules are prepared and packed as usual. The bottle is labelled with the instructions that the patient should add specified amount of freshly boiled and cooled water to granules. The bottle should be shaken well so as to form a homogeneous solution. The label should also carry the storage conditions and time limit in which the reconstituted preparation should be consumed.

Marketed Granules

1. Antepar granules [Burroughs Wellcome (India) Ltd., Bombay - 400023].
   Each contains:
   Piperazine citrate equivalent to 4.5 gm of piperazine hexahydrate and cal. sennosides equ. to 12 mg of sennosides A & B.
2. Calcirol granules (Cadila Labs Ltd., Ahmedabad - 380050).
   Each gm contains:
   Vitamin D_3 60,000 I.U.
3. Flush granules (Dey's Medical Stores, Calcutta - 700087).
   Each 5 gm contains:

Isabgul husk	3.25 gm
Baked bael	0.9 gm
Myrobalan	0.2 gm
Guar gum	0.35 gm

4. Protinex granules (Pfizer Ltd., Bombay - 400021).
   Multivitamin preparation.
5. Alprovit granules (Alkem Labs Ltd., Bombay - 400018).
   Multivitamin preparation.

Marketed Dry Syrups

1. Amfimox dry syrup [Toshniwal Drugs & Pharmaceuticals (P) Ltd., New Delhi - 110002].
   Each 5 ml contains:
   Amoxycillin   125 mg.
2. Ampark dry syrup [Parke-Davis (India) Ltd., Bombay - 400025].
   Each 5 ml contains:
   Ampicillin   125 mg.
3. Ceff dry syrup (Lupin Labs Ltd., Bombay - 400098).
   Each 5 ml contains:
   Cephalexin 125 mg, 250 mg.

4. E-mycin granules (Themis Pharmaceuticals, Bombay - 400093).
   Each 5 ml contains:
   Erythromycin   100 mg.
5. Moxydil dry syrup (Duphar-Interfran Ltd., Bombay - 400018).
   Each 5 ml contains:
   Amoxycillin trihydrate 125 mg, 250 mg.
6. Penmix dry syrup (Deepharma Ltd., New Delhi - 110020).
   Each 3 gm contains:
   Ampicillin   125 mg
   Cloxacillin   125 mg

EFFERVESCENT GRANULES

Effervescent granules are the specially prepared solid dosage form of medicament, meant for internal use. They usually contain a soluble medicinal agent mixed with citric acid, tartaric acid, and sodium bicarbonate. Before administration they are suspended, dissolved in water or are mixed with soft drinks. On mixing with water the carbon dioxide is released as a result of acid-base reaction producing effervescence and the mixture is taken while effervescing. The carbonated water produced from the release of carbon dioxide serves to mask the saline and bitter taste of drugs and the carbon dioxide is said to stimulate the flow of gastric juice and accelerate absorption of medicament.

Effervescent granules are preferred to effervescent powders in order to decrease the rate of dissolution of the substances upon addition to water. Further, if powders are used there may be violent and uncontrollable effervescence with loss of carbon dioxide and ultimately the carbonation of solution may decrease to a great extent.

Method of Preparation

The ingredients used for the preparation of effervescent granules consist of sodium bicarbonate, citric acid, tartaric acid and sodium acid phosphate. Sodium acid phosphate is commonly used in commercial preparations because it is more economical than organic acids. Sodium bicarbonate is used to react with acids when the preparation is added to water, leading to evolution of carbon dioxide. The quantity of the acids used is slightly more than the quantity actually required for complete neutralization of sodium bicarbonate because the preparation with slightly acidic taste are more palatable. The tartaric acid is anhydrous whereas citric acid contains one molecule of water of crystallization which is liberated during heating and serves as a moistening agent for the powders during granulation.

$$3NaHCO_3 + C_6H_8O_7 . H_2O = C6H5Na3O7 + 3CO2 + 3H2O$$
       (Citric acid)   (Sodium citrate)

$$2NaHCO_3 + C_4H_6O_6 = C_4H_4Na_2O_6 + 2CO_2 + 2H_2O$$
       (Tartaric acid) (Sodium tartrate)

Citric acid and tartaric acid both are used because if citric acid alone is used it contains one molecule of water of crystallization which is liberated on heating, will make the mass too wet which will be difficult to pass through the sieve. If tartaric acid alone is used, it is anhydrous and some non-solvent liquid would have to be used for the preparation of granules, otherwise the resulting granules would not be firm but will crumble readily and give salty taste. Moreover citric acid partially neutralizes sodium bicarbonate, the rest of sodium bicarbonate is neutralized by tartaric acid, the slight excess of which imparts acidic taste to the preparation. So relative proportions of citric acid and tartaric acid are based on quantity of water needed to make the powder coherent.

There are two methods of preparation of effervescent granules.

1. Heat method
2. Wet method.

1. Heat Method

A large porcelain or stainless steel evaporating dish is placed over water bath which is being heated to boiling point and must ensure that the evaporating dish is hot when the powders are added to it, failing to do so will not provide sufficient water needed for granulation which will be liberated by citric acid on heating. If the dish will not be hot when the powders are added, it will heat up slowly and the liberated water of crystallization will go on evaporating simultaneously and at no time sufficient water will be available to effect granulation. The water needed for granulation is provided from two sources: (i) from water of crystallization of citric acid which is liberated during heating; and (ii) the water produced from the reactions of citric acid and tartaric acid with sodium bicarbonate.

The powdered ingredients are passed through a sieve no. 60, weighed and mixed. Then they are placed in the dish already warmed on water bath and pressed down with a spatula until the mixture has formed a loose cake or a damp coherent mass is formed. The damp mass is then pressed down a sieve to prepare the granules and dried by keeping in an oven at a temperature not exceeding 60°C. They are packed in dry, wide mouth air-tight containers.

Formula for the preparation of 40 gm of Citro-tartrate of soda effervescent granular base:

Sodium bicarbonate powder	20.40 gm
Tartaric acid powder	10.80 gm
Citric acid powder	7.20 gm
Refined sugar powder	6.00 gm

The method of preparation is described in the above paragraph.

Loss of weight occurs during granulation from two factors:

(a) Loss of moisture by evaporation from the damp mixture.

(b) Loss of carbon dioxide in the above reactions.

These losses constitute approximately one-seventh of the weight of powder used and must be taken into consideration while calculating the amount of granules to be prepared.

2. Wet Method

In the wet method, the mixed ingredients are moistened with a suitable liquid (for which alcohol is the most suitable) in a dish in which alcohol is added in small portions with continuous stirring until a coherent mass is formed. The mass is then passed through a no. 6 sieve and the granules dried at a temperature not exceeding 60°C. The dried granules are again passed through the sieve to break the lumps which may have formed during drying, then they are packed in wide mouth air-tight containers.

Marketed Effervescent Powders

1. Eno fruit salt (Smith Kline Beecham, Nabha - 147201, Punjab).
2. Cetri-soda [Abbot Labs (India) Ltd., Bombay - 400070].
3. Rhino (Mehta Unani Pharmacy & Co., Rajkot - 360001, Gujarat).

Marketed Effervescent Tablets

1. Pepfiz (Ranbaxy Labs Ltd., Delhi - 110020).

BULK POWDERS

They are supplied in bulk quantities and the patient measures out the dose according to his need. The bulk powders meant for internal use are supplied in wide-mouthed containers in which a teaspoon can be entered for easy removal of the contents. Only the nonpotent substances are supplied as bulk powders, e.g., antacids, laxatives, etc.

Bulk powders meant for external application like antiseptic and dusting powders are supplied in cardboard, glass or plastic containers, which are often designed for the specific method of application. The dusting powders are preferably supplied in perforated or sifter top containers.

Rx

Calcium carbonate	37.5 gm
Heavy magnesium carbonate	37.5 gm
Sodium bicarbonate	12.5 gm
Bismuth carbonate	12.5 gm

Make a powder.
Label: The Compound Bismuth Powder. Send 50 gm.
Sig: 5 gm bis in die sumenda.
Type: Bulk powder.

Rx

Rhubarb, in powder	25.0 gm
Ginger, in powder	10.0 gm
Light magnesium carbonate	32.5 gm
Heavy magnesium carbonate	32.5 gm

Make powder.
Label: The Gregory's powder (Compound Rhubarb powder). Send 25 gm.
Directions: 0.5 to 5.0 gm to be taken twice in a day.
Type: Bulk oral powder.

DUSTING POWDERS

Dusting powders are meant for external application to the skin for antiseptic, antipruritic, astringent, antiperspirant, absorbent, protective and lubricant purposes. These powders must be homogenous and in a very fine state of subdivision to enhance effectiveness and minimise local irritation. For this purpose they may be passed through a sieve no.

120. Additionally the dusting powders should flow easily, spread uniformly and stick to the skin when applied. They must be able to protect the skin from irritation caused by friction, moisture or chemical irritants.

Dusting powders are generally prepared by mixing two or more than two ingredients in which starch, kaolin or talc is used as one of the ingredients of formulation. Starch being a carbohydrate can support bacterial growth therefore rarely used. Talcum and other similar substances though are chemically inert substances but are readily contaminated with microorganisms like clostridium tetani, cl. welchii and bacillus anthracis. Therefore they must be sterilized before using in the formulation otherwise they may be a source of infection.

The dusting powders are dispensed in sifter-top containers or pressure aerosols. The pressure aerosol containers are costlier than other containers but can protect the powder from atmospheric conditions and help in the easy application of the preparation. Dusting powders may also be applied with powder puff, a soft brush or a sterile gauze pad but care must be taken to avoid mechanical irritation to the skin surface.

Though the dusting powders are considered non-toxic but the inhalation of light, fluffy powders may lead to pulmonary inflammation of lungs in infants and absorption of boric acid through the broken skin may cause toxic reactions in infants. Therefore proper care must be taken while using these types of preparations.

Rx

Purified talc, sterilised	50 gm
Starch, in powder	25 gm
Zinc oxide	25 gm

Label: Zinc, Starch and Talc dusting powder.
Type: Dusting powder.

Theory

This preparation contains talc which is mineral ingredient and may be contaminated with spores of clostridium tetani and clostridium welchii (a source of tetanus). Therefore whenever talc and kaolin is to be used in dusting powders, must be sterilised by heating at 160°C for one hour to remove these microorganisms. Purified talc has excellent flow and lubricant properties therefore is used in a number of dusting powders.

Starch acts as an absorbent. Zinc oxide acts as an antiseptic and absorbs moisture.

Boric acid should no longer be used in dusting powders since it has been found that it may be absorbed in large amounts through the open skin leading to toxic reactions.

Procedure

Weigh the required quantities of purified talc, sterilised; starch, in powder and zinc oxide. Mix zinc oxide with starch, incorporate purified talc, sterilized. Mix thoroughly. Pass the mixed powders through a sieve no. 120 to remove gritty particles. After sifting, whole of the powder must again be lightly mixed. Pack the powder in sifter-top containers to protect it from air, moisture and contamination as well as convenience of application.

Marketed Dusting Powders

1. Cibazol dusting powder (Hindustan Ciba-Geigy Ltd., Bombay - 400020).

   Contains:
   Sulphathiazole   20% w/w
2. Nebasulf dusting powder (Pfizer Ltd., Bombay - 400021).

   Each gm contains:
   Neomycin sulphate   5 mg
   Bacitracin   250 units
   Sulphacetamide   60 mg
3. Neobacid sprinkling powder [Roland Pharmaceuticals, Berhampur, Distt. Ganjam (Orissa) - 760009].

   Each gm contains:
   Neomycin sulphate   5 mg
   Bacitracin   250 units
   Sulphacetamide   60 mg
4. Salicylic acid compound dusting powder (Alpine Industries, New Delhi - 110028).

   Each contains:
   Salicylic acid   1.5 gm
   Boric acid   2.5 gm
   Purified talc to   50.0 gm

5. Boric talc dusting powder (Alpine Industries, New Delhi - 110028).
   Each contains:

Boric acid	2.5 gm
Starch	5.0 gm
Purified talc to	50.0 gm

INSUFFLATIONS

These are the finely divided powders meant for introduction into the body cavities such as ears, nose, tooth sockets and vagina with the help of an apparatus known as insufflator. This divides the powder into a stream of finely divided particles to the site of application. The major difficulty in using this apparatus is that (i) it is difficult to obtain a measured quantity of drug to get a uniform dose; (ii) it has a tendency to get blocked when the powders used are wet or the apparatus itself is wet. The introduction of newer pressure aerosols have eliminated these difficulties. This method has the advantage that a measured quantity of dose through metered valves is supplied and the product is also protected.

In insufflations the particle size must be very small and they should be absolutely free from irritant and sensitizing effects.

SNUFFS

Snuffs are the finely divided solid dosage form of medicament which are inhaled into the nostrils for their antiseptic, decongestion or bronchodialator action. Snuffs should be dispensed in flat metal boxes with hinged lid.

DENTIFRICES

Dentifrices are the substances which are generally used with the help of tooth brush for cleaning the surfaces of the teeth. They are available in the form of fine powders and pastes.

For the preparation of tooth powders the same general principles already described for mixing the powders are applied. It is important to obtain the cleansing action chiefly by the detergent properties of the powder rather than through the use of harmful abrasives. A mild degree of abrasion is desirable which may be obtained by using chiefly finely precipitated calcium carbonate, one or more of the dibasic calcium phosphate, calcium sulphate, magnesium carbonate, sodium bicarbonate and sodium chloride. They also contain flavours and soap. Tooth pastes contain liquids such as glycerin, sorbitol, water and alcohol. A thickening agent like starch, tragacanth and cellulose derivatives is also incorporated. The sweetening agent added may be sugar but non-carbohydrate sweetening agents are preferred. Saccharin is generally used for this purpose.

The use of strong abrasive substances is harmful because it may damage the tooth structure. Similarly the dentifrices used by the dentist for cleaning purposes should not be used daily, it may spoil the teeth.

Rx

Hard soap in fine powder	5 gm
Precipitated calcium carbonate	93.5 gm
Saccharin sodium	0.3 gm
Clove oil	0.5 ml
Sod. lauryl sulphate	0.7 gm
Make a tooth powder.	

Marketed Medicated Tooth Powders

1. Clinso-Dent (ICPA Health Products Pvt. Ltd., Ankleshwar - 393002).
2. Fixon flavoured denture (ICPA Health Products Pvt. Ltd., Ankleshwar - 393002).
3. Steradent denture cleansing powder (Reckitt & Colman, Calcutta - 700071).

Marketed Medicated Tooth Pastes

1. Emoform (Dentifrices, Trithala - 679534).
   Contains:
   Formalin in a pleasantly flavoured base.
2. Desent tooth paste (Indoco Remedies Ltd., Bombay - 400093).
   Contains:
   Stronium chloride 10% in a dentifrice base.
3. Mentadent G (Hindustan Lever Ltd., Bombay - 400020).
4. Senolin (Warren Pharmaceutical Pvt. Ltd., Bombay - 400058).
5. Sensoform (Warren Pharmaceutical Pvt. Ltd., Bombay - 400058).

CACHETS

Cachets are the solid unit dosage form of medicament in which the drug is enclosed in a tasteless sheet made by pouring a mixture of rice flour and water between two hot, polished, revolving cylinders. The water evaporates and a sheet of wafer is formed known as cachets. Cachets are also known as wafer capsules or capsula amylacea. These are used to enclose nauseous or disagreeable powders and can hold 0.2 to 1.5 gm of powder. Sodium aminosalicylate which is given in a dose of 12 gm daily in the treatment of tuberculosis is commonly prescribed in cachets.

Cachets are hard to swallow as such therefore before administration a cachet should be dipped in water for a few seconds and then placed on the tongue and swallowed with a draught of water. In this way the outer shell of the cachet is softened but the enclosed powder will remain intact. After swallowing, the cachet will disintegrate and the powder will be released.

Advantages

1. They are easy to prepare because no complicated machinery is required (as compared to tablets).
2. Drugs can be extemporaneously and quickly dispensed in cachets.
3. Comparatively large doses of drugs can be dispensed because once they have been softened by dipping in water, even large sizes can be swallowed easily (compared to large size hard capsules).
4. They disintegrate quickly in the stomach.

Disadvantages

1. They are easily damaged.
2. They do no protect the enclosed drugs from light and moisture.
3. They require moistening before swallowing.
4. They cover more space than the corresponding sizes of capsules or tablets.
5. The contents of cachets cannot be greatly compressed because of the fragile nature of the shells.
6. They cannot be filled by large-scale machinery.

Due to these disadvantages cachets are not very commonly used as that of capsules and tablets.

Types of Cachets

There are two types of cachets: (a) wet seal cachets which are sealed by moistening the edges with water; and (b) dry seal cachets which do not require any moisture for sealing.

(a) Wet Seal Cachets

A wet seal cachet is made up of two similar convex halves having flat edges. The weighed amount of powder is placed in one half, the edges of the other half are moistened with water and placed exactly over the first half containing the powder. The flat edges of both the halves are pressed together so that a perfect seal is made and the powder is completely enclosed.

Wet Seal Cachet Machine

This machine consists of three thin metal plates joined by hinges so that they may be opened or superposed as and when desired. The halves of the cachet in which the powder is to be filled are placed in the central plate where they fit loosely. The second plate having the corresponding holes like that of first plate is then superposed on the central plate. The object of this plate is to protect the edges of cachets while they are being filled. The powder is filled in the halves placed in first plate, by means of funnels supplied with the machine. The powder so filled is then pressed down with a small plunger or metal thimble also supplied with the machine.

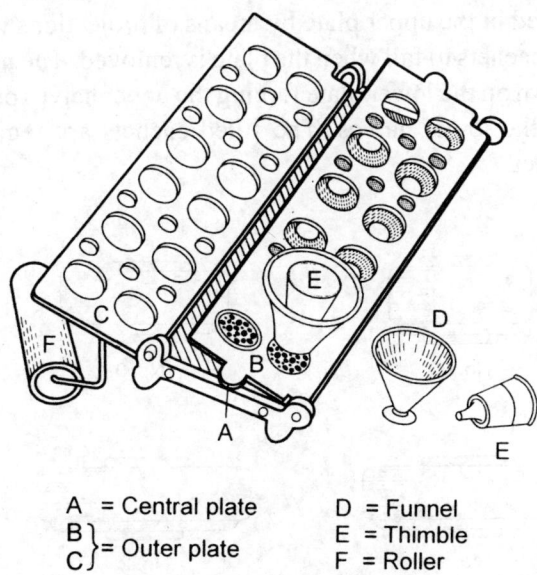

A = Central plate   D = Funnel
B }= Outer plate   E = Thimble
C }   F = Roller

Fig. 10.1. Cachet machine.

After filling the lower halves, the second plate is folded back to its original position. The other halves of the cachets are then placed in the corresponding holes of the third plate. The edges of these halves are then moistened with water from a roller attached with the machine. This plate is turned over the central plate in such a way that the edges of two halves completely cover each other and little pressure is applied so as to join the two halves. The upper plate is then lifted upward which will bring the complete cachets with it. The finished cachets are gently removed from upper plate and securely packed in cardboard or tin boxes. Cachets should be labelled with directions for administration, e.g., "Immerse in water for a few seconds and then swallow with a draught of water.".

(b) Dry Seal Cachets

Dry seal cachets consists of two halves, the upper half and the lower half, the former is little larger in diameter. The powder is filled in lower half and upper half is fitted over it like a lid on a box. The backs of upper as well as lower halves have small projections which are used to fix the cachet in the holes of the machine. The lower halves are fitted into the lower plate of the machine and powder filled therein. The upper halves are fitted in the upper plate by means of projections which will not allow the cachets to fall when the plate is removed. The upper plate is pressed down on the lower plate forcing the upper halves or lids to fit exactly over the lower halves. The filled cachets are removed and packed in boxes.

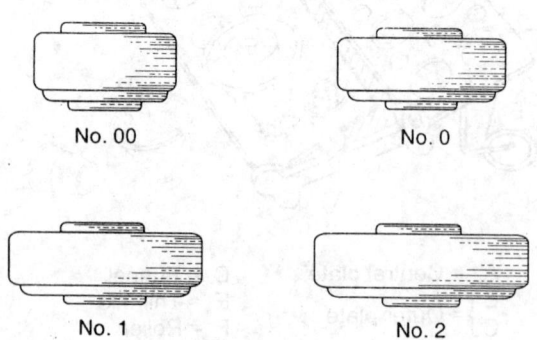

No. 00   No. 0

No. 1   No. 2

Fig. 10.2. Dry seal cachets.

The dry seal cachets have advantages that there are no chances of escaping the powder and can be prepared more quickly and are more hygienic.

Dispensing

The catchets are dispensed in boxes or tins in which they are packed on their edges or lying flat. If necessary the compartments may be filled with cotton wool. Catchets should be labelled with directions for its use: "Immerse in water for a few seconds and then swallow with a draught of water.".

MOLDED TABLETS

1. Hypodermic tablets
2. Dispensing tablets.

Molded Tablets or Tablet Triturates "TT"

Molded tablets are small disk-shaped tablets which are prepared by forcing the soft mass into the cavities of the mold. Generally potent medicaments and highly toxic drugs in small doses are used for preparing the molded tablets. The potent medicament is diluted with a diluent like lactose, dextrose, sucrose, or a mixture of lactose and sucrose. The mixed powders are moistened with a suitable dilution of alcohol (generally

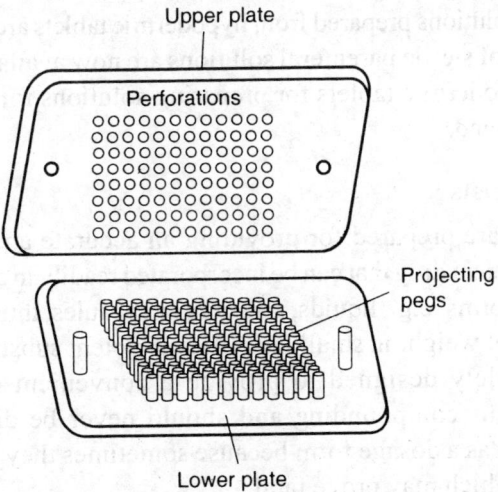

Fig. 10.3. Mold for preparing molded tablets.

50% alcohol is used) and mixed thoroughly so as to get a soft mass. The soft mass so prepared is pressed into the perforations of the mold with a spatula. The excess of the mass is removed by applying pressure over the spatula. This perforated plate having exactly the same number of projecting pegs as that of perforations and these projecting pegs completely fit into the holes. A little pressure is applied over the top plate which will force the plate move downward, leaving the molded tablets on the projecting pegs. The ejected tablets are spread in single layers on clean surface and dried either by keeping in warm place or hot air oven.

Now a days tablet triturates may also be prepared on automatic tablet triturate machines including tablet making machines. A tablet triturate machine can prepare 2500 tablet triturates per minute.

Hypodermic Tablets

Hypodermic tablets are soft, readily soluble tablets which are made in a tablet triturate mold. They are used for preparing solutions to be injected, therefore in selecting the materials used for preparing the hypodermic tablets care must be taken that they should be completely and readily soluble and no insoluble particle should be present. They should be free from bacterial contamination and proper precautions should be taken during molding regarding contamination and cleanliness.

Since the solutions prepared from hypodermic tablets are rarely sterile and a number of sterile parenteral solutions are now available therefore the use of hypodermic tablets for preparing solutions for injections is being discouraged.

Dispensing Tablets

These tablets are prepared for providing an accurate and convenient quantity of a potent drug that can be incorporated readily in compounding other dosage forms, e.g., liquids, powders or capsules, thus eliminating the necessity of weighing small quantities of potent substances. These tablets are solely designed to provide a convenient quantity for extemporaneous compounding and should never be dispensed for administration as a dosage form because sometimes they contain very potent drugs which may prove fatal.

MONOPHASIC LIQUID DOSAGE FORMS

A solution is a clear, homogeneous mixture that is prepared by dissolving a solid, liquid or gas in another liquid. The component of a solution present in large amount is known as solvent and the component present in lesser amount is known as solute. A solution is homogeneous because the solute is in a molecular or ionic state of subdivision, therefore, a true solution is a one phase system. Solutions may be used internally or applied externally whereas mixtures are meant for oral administration. Mixtures are mainly prescribed for acute conditions such as cough, indigestion, diarrhoea, constipation and rheumatism. They are prepared extemporaneously and supplied only for a few days treatment because if they are stored for more than a few weeks even under normal conditions they may deteriorate.

Advantages

1. They are homogeneous, therefore the medicament is uniformly distributed throughout the liquid.
2. The doses can be easily adjusted according to the need of the patient.
3. They can be easily measured with the household measures.
4. They are more quickly effective than tablets or capsules because they are already in the solution form and absorption starts quickly.
5. Some drugs like potassium iodide and bromide leads to gastric pain if taken in the tablet or capsule form but this pain may be reduced when these drugs are administered in the solution form because of dilution factor.
6. They can be easily coloured, flavoured or sweetened.
7. Children or patients who cannot swallow tablets or capsules can easily ingest solutions.
8. There are certain drugs which can only be administered in liquid dosage form, e.g., castor oil and liquid paraffin, etc.

Disadvantages

1. They are difficult to carry and there are chances of breakage of container with the complete loss of contents.
2. In some medicaments their unpleasant taste and flavour is difficult to mask.
3. They are less stable as compared to solid dosage forms because deterioration is faster in solutions.

SOLUBILITY

When an excess of a solid is brought in contact with the solvent and the solid is allowed to dissolve in the solvent, after some time a stage is reached when an equilibrium is established between the solute and the solvent and no more solute dissolves, the resulting solution is said to be saturated at that temperature and the extent to which the solute dissolves is known as its solubility. A solution is said to be supersaturated when it contains a larger amount of the solute than is necessary to form a saturated solution at a particular temperature. These supersaturated solutions create formulation problems because they deposit the excess of substance upon standing and lead to undesirable results. Temperature of 20°C is considered the optimum temperature for the preparation of stable saturated solutions because this is the room temperature at which the medicines are supposed to be kept and used.

Most substances whether solid, liquid or gas can be dissolved in some liquid but none is soluble in all liquids, some of them may be poorly soluble, slightly soluble, highly soluble or even may be insoluble. Water is always considered the most suitable vehicle for the preparation of liquid formulations but a large number of modern drugs are insoluble in it. Hence the solubility of most of these compounds can be increased by one or more of the following methods:

1. Solubilization
2. Co-solvency
3. Complexation
4. Hydrotrophy
5. Chemical modification of the drug
6. pH adjustments.

1. Solubilization

Solubilization is the process in which the water insoluble substances are dissolved in aqueous solutions in the presence of surfactants. The mechanism for this phenomenon is that the surface active agents when added to the solution to be formed tend to aggregate in groups of 100-150 molecules known as micelles. This phenomenon occurs at a certain concentration of surfactant which is known as critical micelle concentration or CMC. Solubilization occurs either by dissolving the solute in the micelle or the solute is adsorbed on to the micelle. Thus the solubilization starts at critical micelle concentration and generally increases with increase in the concentration of micelles.

The solutions so formed are thermodynamically stable. Hence the phenomenon of solubilization is widely used in the development of pharmaceutical formulations. Many water-insoluble drugs are formulated as clear, aqueous solutions by the process of miceller solubilization. A number of drugs can be solubilized in a variety of solvents by using different surface active agents. The examples of drugs which can be solubilized are: fat soluble vitamins A, D, E & K; antibiotics like chloramphenicol, griseofulvin and amphotericin B; analgesics like aspirin, acetanilide and phenacetin, etc. Many alkaloids and glycosides are also solubilized in this way.

2. Co-Solvency

The solubility of poorly soluble drugs in water can be increased by mixing it with some water miscible solvent in which the drug is readily soluble. This phenomenon is known as co-solvency and the solvents used in combination to increase the solubility of the solute are known as co-solvents. Most of the solvent mixtures consist of water, alcohol, glycerin, propylene glycol and syrups.

3. Complexation

Insoluble substances often react with a soluble ingredient to form a complex which is readily soluble in water. A very common example of this type is the formation of tri-iodide complex when iodine and potassium iodide are mixed together. Iodine is insoluble in water whereas the tri-iodide complex so formed is readily soluble in water. The solubility of caffeine is 1:50 whereas the solubility of caffeine and sodium benzoate is 1:1.2 in water. When the solubility is increased by complexation, one has to make sure that the complex formed is reversible, dissociates easily and releases the active ingredients readily otherwise the active ingredient becomes therapeutically ineffective.

4. Hydrotrophy

The term hydrotrophy refers to the increase in solubility of insoluble or slightly soluble drugs in water by the addition of additives, which are not surface active agents. The exact mechanism by which this effect occurs is not clear. The mechanism might be a solubilization, complexation, co-solvency or a combination of several factors. The phenomenon has very little use in pharmaceutical systems.

5. Chemical Modification of the Drug

Many drugs which are poorly soluble in water can be chemically converted into their derivatives which are appreciably soluble in water. For example, alkaloids are poorly soluble in water whereas alkaloidal salts are freely soluble in water. Similarly many other drugs like corticosteroids, etc., can be converted into water soluble derivatives. This approach is highly successful in certain types of drugs but has several practical limitations.

6. pH Adjustments

The solubilities of chemotherapeutic agents which are weak acids or weak bases can be markedly influenced by variations in pH. However, this is not always the best course of action. Before adjusting the pH of any preparation, numerous other implications must also be taken into consideration which may markedly affect the stability of the preparation.

Other Formulation Problems

It is not sufficient to formulate a liquid dosage form that has the desired concentrations of the active ingredients, pH, colour, taste and flavour but should also be chemically and physically stable. The chemical stability of the active ingredients of the formulation are of primary importance and the formulation should be designed to minimize hydrolysis, oxidation, reduction, polymerization or any other chemical change of the active ingredients. Instability also includes variation in colour, flavours, cloudiness or precipitation, bacterial growth, viscosity decrease, etc. Caking of suspensions or cracking of emulsions also leads to instability of preparations. Because of these problems it is difficult to prepare liquid dosage forms with an extended stability, therefore many drugs are prepared in the form of powders which are required to be dissolved in a suitable vehicle immediately before its use.

Liquid preparations which are to be administered into the eyes or meant for parenteral administration must be sterile and they should be isotonic with the lacrymal secretions or blood serum as the case may be. Oral preparations should be elegant in appearance, colour, flavour, taste, etc. They should possess the desirable viscosity as regards to pourability, stability and effectiveness.

LIQUID FORMULATIONS FOR INTERNAL USE

Mixtures

A mixture is a liquid preparation intended for oral administration in which drug or drugs are dissolved, suspended or dispersed in a suitable vehicle and generally several doses are contained in a bottle. When only one dose is dispensed it is known as draught.

Mixtures differ from solutions that the mixtures may be homogeneous or heterogeneous and are for oral administration whereas solutions are homogeneous and are for external or internal use. Mixtures are extemporaneously prepared and they are supplied in such doses that whole of the mixture is used up within a few days. If need arises then fresh mixture is prepared.

Advantages of Mixtures

1. They are more quickly effective than solid dosage forms which require previous disintegration in the body before absorption can take place.
2. Certain substances can only be given in liquid form because they are inconvenient to administer in any other form due to their liquid nature and large dose, e.g., castor oil, liquid paraffin, aromatic waters, etc.
3. Certain substances like potassium iodide and potassium bromide may cause pain in the stomach if given in the solid form as a powder or a tablet.
4. Certain substances are useful when they are administered in a suspension form, e.g., light kaolin and bismuth salts, because in suspension form they afford large surface area for the absorption of toxic substances in the gut.
5. Mixtures are easy to administer and economical as compared to other oral preparations.

Disadvantages

1. They are comparatively less stable than solid dosage forms.
2. Incompatibility is more in liquid preparations as compared to solid ones.
3. They are more bulky and difficult to carry.

Classification

Mixtures may be classified as follows:

1. Simple mixtures
2. Mixtures containing diffusible solids
3. Mixtures containing indiffusible solids
4. Mixtures containing precipitate forming liquids
5. Mixtures containing slightly soluble liquids
6. Miscellaneous mixtures.

Simple Mixtures

A simple mixture is one which contains only soluble ingredients, e.g., carminative mixture, diaphoretic mixture, cough expectorant, etc.

Method of Dispensing

(a) Dissolve the solid substances in 3/4 th of the vehicle. The reasons for this is that (i) the volume occupied by the other ingredients rarely exceeds the remaining 1/4 th, but if this volume exceeds, the 3/4 th quantity of vehicle used must be reduced; (ii) solution formation is hastened by using as much of the solvent as convenient.

(b) Examine the solution critically by holding the container against light. If foreign particles are visible pass the solution through cotton wool, further pour little more vehicle over cotton wool so that the solution therein is removed.

(c) Add any liquid ingredients. Volatile liquids are added at the end just before adjusting the final volume with vehicle.

(d) Add more of vehicle to produce the final volume.

(e) Transfer the mixture to a bottle, cork, and thoroughly polish the bottle to remove finger prints. Attach the label, wrap the bottle and dispense.

Mixtures containing diffusible solids and indiffusible solids are discussed under suspensions.

Marketed Mixtures/Liquid Preparations

1. Carminative mixture (Zandu Pharmaceutical Works Ltd., Bombay - 400025).
   Each contains:
   Sodium bicarbonate, Spt. ammonia aromatic, Tr. gentian comp., Tr. card. comp., Spt. chloroform, Tr. zingiberis.
2. Gelusil liquid (Warner-Hindustan Division, Bombay - 400072).
   Each 5 ml contains:

Magnesium trisilicate	625 mg
Dried aluminium hydroxide gel	312 mg

3. Kaolin mixture (Arora Pharmaceuticals Pvt. Ltd., New Delhi - 110035).

Each 15 ml contains:

Light kaolin	2 mg
Light mag. carbonate	0.6 gm
Sodium bicarbonate	0.6 gm
Peppermint water	15 ml

4. Kloratum liquid (Klar Sehen Pvt. Ltd., Calcutta - 700026).

Each 5 ml contains:
Pot. chloride   500 mg

5. Lederplex liquid (Cyanamid India Ltd., Lederle Division, Bombay - 400025).

Marketed Solutions

1. Acriflavine solution (Agrawal Pharmaceuticals, Delhi - 110092).

Each ml contains:
Acriflavine   0.1%

2. Cetrimide HC 0.5% liquid (I.C.I. India Ltd., Madras - 600008).

Contains:

Cetrimide	0.5% w/w
Chlorhexidine HCl	0.1% w/w

3. Dettol antiseptic liquid (Reckitt & Colman of India Ltd., Calcutta - 700071).

Contains:

Chloroxylenol	4.8% w/v
Terpineol	9% v/v
Absolute alcohol	13.1% v/v

4. Merbromin solution (Agrawal Pharmaceuticals, Delhi - 110092).

Contains:
Merbromin   2%

5. Savlon hospital concentrate liquid (I.C.I. India Ltd., Madras - 600008).

Contains:

Chlorhexidine gluconate	7.5% v/v
Cetrimide	15% w/w

SYRUPS

Syrups are the sweet, viscous, concentrated aqueous solutions of sucrose or other sugars in water or any other suitable aqueous vehicle. When purified water alone is used in making the solution of sucrose the preparation is known as syrup or simple syrup. When the preparation contains some medicinal substance it is known as medicated syrup. When the syrup does not contain any medicament but contains various aromatic or pleasantly flavoured substances are known as flavouring syrups. They are used for masking the disagreeable taste of bitter or saline drugs. They are also used as vehicles or flavours for extemporaneous preparations.

In addition to sucrose, certain other polyols, such as glycerin, sorbitol or other polyhydric alcohols may be added in small amounts to retard crystallization of sucrose or to increase the solubility of other added ingredients.

In the manufacture of syrups the sucrose and purified water free from foreign substances should be selected and clean containers must be used to avoid contamination during preparation. Dilute solutions of sucrose support mold, yeast and other microbial growth whereas the growth of such microorganisms is usually retarded when the concentration of sucrose is 65% weight by weight or more but a saturated solution may lead to crystallization of sucrose.

Only small quantities of syrups should be prepared which can be used within a few months. If large quantities are to be prepared then they must be preserved well to prevent contamination. Syrups can be well preserved at a temperature not exceeding 25°C. In dilute solutions preservatives like glycerin, methyl paraben, benzoic acid and sodium benzoate may be added.

Now a days artificial syrups prepared from artificial sweetening agents are available in the market. They have the advantage over syrups prepared from sugars that they do not contain any carbohydrate therefore can be easily given to diabetic patients. Moreover they have lesser stability problems than sugar-based syrups.

Examples are syrup, orange syrup, tolu syrup, raspberry syrup, black currant syrup and wild cherry syrup.

Storage: Syrups should be stored in a well-closed container and at a temperature not exceeding 30°C.

Marketed Syrups

1. Benadryl syrup [Parke-Davis (India) Ltd., Bombay - 400025].
   Each 5 ml contains:
   Diphenhydramine HCl   12.5 mg
2. Corex cough syrup (Pfizer Ltd., Bombay - 400021).
   Each 5 ml contains:
   Chlorpheniramine maleate   4 mg
   Codein phos.   10 mg
   Ephedrine HCl   5 mg
   Sod. citrate   150 mg
   Menthol   0.1 mg
3. Crocin syrup (Duphar-Interfran Ltd., Bombay - 400018).
   Each 5 ml contains:
   Paracetamol   125 mg
4. Metacin syrup (Themis Pharmaceuticals, Bombay - 400093).
   Each 5 ml contains:
   Paracetamol   0.125 gm
5. Polybion syrup [E. Merck (India) Ltd., Bombay - 400018].
   Multivitamin preparation.
6. Sudafed syrup [Burroughs Wellcome (India) Ltd., Bombay - 400023].
7. Ultragin syrup (Geoffrey Manners & Co. Ltd., Bombay - 400038).
   Each 5 ml contains:
   Analgin   15.62 mg
   Paracetamol   15.62 mg
8. Vi-Syneral syrup [U.S. Vitamin (India) Ltd., Bombay - 400018].
   Multivitamin preparation.

ELIXIRS

Elixirs are clear, pleasantly flavoured, sweetened hydroalcoholic liquid preparations for oral administration. The main ingredients of elixirs are ethanol and water but glycerin, sorbitol, propylene glycol, flavouring agents, sugar and preservatives may be incorporated to the preparation. The elixirs may be medicated or non-medicated. The medicated elixirs usually contain very potent drugs such as antibiotics, antihistaminics and sedatives. The bitter and nauseous taste of certain drugs can be masked by adding flavouring and sweetening agents. The non-medicated elixirs are used as flavours and vehicles.

Examples are chloral elixir, chlorpheniramine elixir, paracetamol elixir, phenobarbitone elixir, piperazine citrate elixir.

Storage: Since elixirs contain alcohol and usually some volatile oils which deteriorate in the presence of air and light therefore they should be stored in tightly closed, light resistant containers and in a cool place.

Marketed Elixirs

1. Betonin (Vitamin B-Complex) elixir (Boots Pharmaceuticals Ltd., Bombay - 400038).
2. Cadiphylate elixir (Cadila Laboratories Ltd., Ahmedabad - 380050).

   Each 5 ml contains:

Theophylline ethanoate of piperazine	80 mg
Ephedrine HCl	12 mg
Glyceryl guaiacolate ether	50 mg
Phenobarbitone	4 mg
Alcohol	0.55 ml

3. Ephedrine compound elixir [Parke-Davis (India) Ltd., Bombay - 400025].

   Each 5 ml contains:

Ephedrine sulphate	22.80	mg
Caffeine	91.2	mg
Sod. salicylate	114.0	mg
Sod. iodide	60.8	mg
Ext. of belladonna green	14.25	mg
Alcohol	0.787	ml
Alcohol content	15%	v/v

4. Phosfomin tonic elixir (Sarabhai Chemicals, Vadodra - 390007).
5. Phosfomin iron tonic elixir (Sarabhai Chemicals, Vadodra - 390007).
6. Piperazine elixir [Burroughs Wellcome (India) Ltd., Bombay - 400023].
7. Rubraplex elixir (Sarabhai Chemicals, Vadodra - 390007).

LINCTUSES

LInctuses are sweet, viscous liquid preparations usually containing medicinal substances which have demulcent, sedative or expectorant properties. They are used for the treatment of cough. They produce soothening effect on the mucous membrane of the throat. To obtain the maximum effect they should be taken in small doses, sipped and swallowed slowly without the addition of water.

Examples are codeine linctus, noscapine linctus, simple linctus.

Marketed Linctuses

1. Coskin linctus (Warner-Hindustan Division, Bombay - 400072).
   Each 5 ml contains:

Noscapine	15 mg
Glyceryl guaiacolate	100 mg
Chlorpheniramine maleate	2 mg
Spirit chloroform	0.4 ml
Menthol	1 mg
Alcohol content	8-10% v/v

2. Coscopin linctus (Biological E. Ltd., Hyderabad - 500020).
3. Protussa cough linctus (Boots Pharmaceuticals Ltd., Bombay - 400038).
   Each 5 ml contains:

Noscapine	5 mg
Sod. citrate	125 mg
Ephedrine HCl	3 mg
Tinct. belladonna	0.125 ml
Tolu solution	0.133 ml

Marketed Expectorants

1. Avil expectorant (Hoechst India Ltd., Bombay - 400021).
2. Benadryl cough expectorant [Parke-Davis (India) Ltd., Bombay - 400025].
3. Broncare expectorant (Themis Pharmaceuticals, Bombay - 400093).
4. Novadin expectorant (Novus Pharmaceuticals, Bombay - 400093).
5. Piritone Glaxo expectorant (Glaxo India Ltd., Bombay - 400025).
   Each 5 ml contains:

Chlorpheniramine maleate	2.5 mg
Amm. chloride	125.0 mg
Sod. citrate	55.0 mg

DROPS

These are liquid preparations meant for oral administration. Generally potent medicaments and vitamins are formulated as drops. Usually vitamin A and D concentrates in fish liver oil are presented as drops for administration to children. Since these drops contain potent medicaments, the dose must be measured precisely with droppers which are accurately graduated in fractions of a millilitre.

Marketed Drops

1. Abdec drops [Parke-Davis (India) Ltd., Bombay - 400025]. Multivitamin drops.
2. Arovit drops (Roche Products Ltd., Bombay - 400034). Each ml contains:
   Vit. A   150,000 I.U.
3. Crocin drops (Duphar-Interfran Ltd., Bombay - 400018). Each ml contains:
   Paracetamol   150 mg
4. Digiplex drops (Rallis India Ltd., Bombay - 400001). Each ml contains:
   Diastase   31.25 mg
   Pepsin   10.0 mg
5. Incremin drops (Cyanamid India Ltd., Lederle Division, Bombay - 400025). Contains:
   Lysine and vitamins.
6. Metacin drops (Themis Pharmaceuticals, Bombay - 400093).
7. Sporidex drops (Ranbaxy Laboratories Ltd., New Delhi - 110019). Each ml contains:
   Cephalexin   100 mg
8. Vi-Syneral vitamin drops [U.S. Vitamin (India) Ltd., Bombay - 400018]. Multivitamin drops.
9. Toothache drops (Alpine Industries, New Delhi - 110028). Each contains:
   Clove oil   5% w/v
   Methyl salicylate   15% w/v
   Camphor   1% w/v
   Peppermint oil   6% w/v

DRAUGHTS

A draught is a liquid preparation taken as a single dose. If several doses are prescribed they are dispensed in separate containers but Ipecacuanha

Emetic Draught is an exception in which several doses are prescribed in a multiple dose container.

Liquids for External Use

1. Liquids to be used in the mouth and other body cavities, e.g., gargles, mouth washes, throat paints, sprays, enemas, douches, nasal drops, inhalations, eye drops, eye lotions, ear drops, etc.
2. Liquids to be applied to the skin, e.g., liniments, lotions, etc.

1. LIQUIDS TO BE USED IN THE MOUTH AND OTHER BODY CAVITIES

Gargles

Gargles are aqueous solutions used for the treatment of an infection of the throat. Usually they are concentrated solutions and must be diluted with water before use. In using the gargles they are brought into intimate contact with the mucous membrane of the throat and are allowed to remain there for a few moments after which they are thrown out of the mouth.

Gargles should be dispensed in clear, fluted glass bottles closed with a plastic screw cap and labelled in such a way that it clearly distinguishes them from preparations meant for internal administration. If they are to be swallowed after use, they should be dispensed in bottles similar to the bottles used for mixtures. If the gargles are to be protected from light, they should be dispensed in light-resistant containers. Directions should be given on the label for diluting the gargles before use.

Examples are phenol gargles, potassium chlorate and phenol gargles.

Rx

Phenol glycerin	5 ml
Amaranth solution	1 ml
Water	up to 100 ml

Label: The gargles.
Sig: Dilute it with an equal volume of warm water before use.
Type: Gargles.

Procedure

Mix Amaranth solution (1% w/v in chloroform water) with small amount of water, add phenol glycerin (16% w/w phenol and 84% w/w glycerin) and mix. To this incorporate more of vehicle to produce the required volume. Transfer to a container, label and dispense. Secondary label "Not to be swallowed in large amounts" must be attached.

Uses

It is used as gargles for the treatment of pharynx and nasopharynx by forcing air from the lungs through the gargles which is held in the throat.

Phenol gargles should be diluted with an equal volume of warm water before use.

Mouth Washes

A mouth wash is an aqueous solution with a pleasant taste and odour used for rinsing, deodorant, refreshing or antiseptic action. It may contain alcohol, glycerin, sweetening agents, surface active agents, flavouring agents and colouring agents. Medicated mouth washes containing astringents, antibacterial agents, protein precipitants or other agents are also used but they must be used under the supervision of the dentist. A very simple preparation like compound sodium chloride mouth wash containing sodium chloride and sodium bicarbonate in peppermint water is commonly used. The medicated mouth washes should not be indiscriminately used by a normal person, the continuous use may prove harmful.

Mouth washes should be dispensed in clear fluted bottles. The container should be labelled with directions for diluting the mouth wash before use.

Rx

Sodium chloride	2 gm
Sodium bicarbonate	1 gm
Amaranth solution	2 ml
Peppermint water	up to 100 ml

Label: The mouth wash.
Directions:
1. Dilute it with an equal volume of warm water before use.
2. Rinse the mouth 3-4 times daily as required.

Type: Mouth wash.

Procedure

Dissolve the weighed quantities of sodium chloride and sodium bicarbonate in 3/4 th of the vehicle, add Amaranth solution and incorporate more of vehicle to produce the required volume. Transfer to a bottle, label and dispense. The secondary label "Not to be swallowed in large amounts" must be attached.

Uses

Compound sodium chloride mouth wash is a simple mouth wash which is used to cleanse and deodorise the buccal cavity. It is very refreshing particularly to the bed-ridden patients.

1. Sodium chloride makes the preparation isotonic.
2. Sodium bicarbonate can dissolve mucous therefore added to spray solutions and washes for the throat and nose.
3. Amaranth solution is used as a colouring agent.
4. Peppermint water is used to impart pleasant taste and odour to the preparation.

Marketed Mouth-washes and Gargles

1. Dettolin mouth wash and gargles (Reckitt & Colman of India Ltd., Calcutta - 700071).
   Contains:

Chloroxylenol	1.02% w/v
Menthol	0.12% w/v
Absolute alcohol	60.8% v/v

   Amaranth as colour.
2. Garlin mouth-wash (Klar Sehen Pvt. Ltd., Calcutta - 700026).
3. Listrine liquid (Warner-Hindustan Division, Bombay - 400072).
   Contains:

Thymol	0.06% w/v
Eucalyptol	0.09% w/v
Methyl salicylate	0.06% w/v
Menthol	0.04% w/v
Benzoic acid	0.15% w/v
Alcohol	25.27% v/v

4. Thymoral mouth-wash (Rays Labs Pvt. Ltd., Calcutta - 700007).
5. Povidine mouth-wash (Stadmed Pvt. Ltd., Calcutta - 700071).
   Each contains:

Povidone iodine	1% w/v

Throat Paints

Throat paints are viscous liquid preparations used for mouth and throat infections. In general the drugs used are antibiotics, sulphonamides, iodides, phenol and tannic acid. Glycerin is commonly used as a base because of its viscous nature and agreeable taste. Boroglycerin, phenol glycerin, tannic acid glycerin and compound iodine paint (Mandle's paint) are commonly used as throat paints. They are made viscous so that the drug should remain in contact with mucous membrane for sufficiently long time to produce its prolonged action.

Throat paints should be dispensed in airtight, coloured fluted bottles in order to distinguish them from preparations meant of internal use. Such containers should be fitted with glass stoppers or other suitable closures. They should be stored in a cool place. The containers should be labelled with instructions "Not to be swallowed in large amounts".

Marketed Throat Paints

1. Candid mouth paint (Glenmark Pharmaceuticals Ltd., Bombay - 400026).
   Each contains:
   Clotrimazole   1%
2. Dentex gum paint (Dermocare Labs, Ahmedabad - 380001).
   Each contains:

Tannic acid	3%
Pot. iodide	2%
Iodine	0.5%
Thymol	0.2%
Menthol	0.2%
Camphor	0.2%

3. Gumtex gum paint (Arora Pharmaceuticals Pvt. Ltd., New Delhi - 110035).
4. Gum paint (Alpine Industries, New Delhi - 110028).
5. Mastic paint compound (Alpine Industries, New Delhi - 110028).
6. Megenta paint (Alpine Industries, New Delhi - 110028).
7. Paint of iodine compound (Mandle's paint) (Alpine Industries, New Delhi - 110028).
8. Paintex paint (Mendine Pharmaceuticals Pvt. Ltd., Calcutta - 700027).
   Each ml contains:

Clove oil	3%
Camphor	0.1%

Menthol	1%
Glycerin	5%
Iodine tincture	7%
Sol. ether	10%
Peppermint water conc.	15%
Alcohol	56%

Sprays

Throat sprays are the liquid preparations which are sprayed into the mouth for their laryngitis, pharyngitis and tonsillitis action. But mainly they are used to produce their action on the lungs for which they are sprayed with a special type of atomiser known as nebuliser. Adrenaline and atropine spray is used as a bronchodialator in asthma and hay fever.

Sprays should be dispensed in coloured fluted bottles labelled with the instructions "For external use only.".

Marketed Inhaler Sprays

1. Aerocort inhaler (Cipla Ltd., Bombay - 400008).
2. Asthalin inhaler (Cipla Ltd., Bombay - 400008).
   Each metered dose contains:
   Salbutamol sulphate   100 mcg
3. Autohaler inhaler (Cipla Ltd., Bombay - 400008).
4. Beclate inhaler (Cipla Ltd., Bombay - 400008).
5. Cromal-5 inhaler (Cipla Ltd., Bombay - 400008).

Enemas

Enemas are aqueous or oily solutions or suspensions intended for introduction into the rectum for their purgative, sedative, anthelmintic, anti-inflammatory or nutritive effects. They may also be used for x-ray examination of the lower bowel. Among the commonly used drugs in solution form which act as cleansing enemas include isotonic solution of sodium chloride, sodium bicarbonate 2%, sodium phosphate, magnesium sulphate, soap, glycerin and a combination of these substances. The other drugs used in the form of enemas include olive oil, arachis oil, chloral hydrate, paraldehyde, turpentine, alum, tannic acid and barium sulphate, etc.

Usually solutions in volume of 500 ml to 1000 ml, depending on the age and condition of the patient is introduced as enema. However the commercially availably concentrated enemas are introduced in small volumes of 100 to 200 ml. Large volume enemas should be warmed to body temperature before administration.

There are two type of enemas (i) evacuant enemas and (ii) retention enemas. Evacuant enemas may be given up to 2 litres whereas retention enemas do not normally exceed 100 ml in volume.

Disposable Enemas

Now a days enemas are available in disposable plastic bags. Such enemas include magnesium sulphate as evacuant enemas and prednisolone as retention enemas.

A typical example of evacuant enema:

Rx

Soft soap   25 gm
Purified water   500 ml
Label: The soap enema.
Sig: To be used as directed.
Type: Evacuant enema.

Procedure

Dissolve the soft soap in purified water. Transfer to a container, label and dispense. Attach the secondary label "For rectal use only" and dispense.

Uses

It is used as an evacuant enema.

Precaution

Large volume enemas should be warmed to body temperature before administration.

Marketed Medicated Enemas

1. Laxicon enema (Stadmed Pvt. Ltd., Calcutta - 700071).
   Each contains:
   Dioctyl sod. sulphosuccinate   0.25%
2. Practo-Clyss (Comteck Labs, Bombay - 400016).
   Each contains:
   Sod. dihydrogen phosphate   16% w/w
   Sod. phosphate I.P.   6% w/w
   Purified water q.s.

Douches

A douche is an aqueous solution meant for introduction into one of the body cavities either for medicinal treatment or for hygienic purposes. The word 'douche' is most commonly used for vaginal solutions and are generally called irrigations. Douches are also used to irrigate the eyes, ear or nasal cavities for cleaning or removing the foreign particles or discharges from these cavities.

Many douches are dispensed in the form of powders or tablets accompanied by directions for dissolving in a specified quantity of water, usually warm. They are also dispensed as concentrated solutions and the patient is required to dilute it accordingly before use.

Solutions commonly used as cleansing douche include water, sodium chloride (0.2% isotonic), boric acid 2%, sodium bicarbonate 2%. Medicated solutions include mercuric chloride 1: 3000 to 1: 10000, silver nitrate 1: 1000, potassium permanganate 1: 4000 or lactic acid 0.5 to 3%. Weak solutions of tannic acid, acetic acid or vinegar and alum are used as astringents. Potassium permanganate, peroxides or perborates may be used for their deodorizing effect.

The equipment used is known as douche can and consists of a metal or rubber container to hold the solution. To this is attached a rubber tube about 2 metre long fitted with a nozzle, which may be of glass or rubber. Generally 1 litre to 2 litre of solution is used as a douche.

Ear Drops

Ear drops are the liquid preparations in which the drugs are dissolved or suspended in a suitable vehicle like water, dilute alcohol, glycerin, propylene glycol or any other suitable solvent and are intended for instillation into the ear with a dropper. Generally propylene glycol, polyethylene glycol and glycerin are most commonly used vehicles. Water is disfavoured because it would face difficulty in mixing with the secretions of ear which are mainly fatty.

Ear drops are generally used for cleansing the ear, drying weeping surfaces, softening the wax and for treating the mild infections.

Ear drops are dispensed in coloured fluted bottles attached with a dropper or in suitable plastic containers. The containers should be labelled "For external use only.".

Rx

Sodium bicarbonate   5 gm
Glycerin   30 ml
Purified water, freshly boiled and cooled to 100 ml
Label: The ear drops.
Sig: 2-3 drops to be put into each ear as directed.
Type: Ear drops.

Procedure

Dissolve the sodium bicarbonate in about 60 ml of purified water, add the glycerin and sufficient purified water to produce the required volume, mix thoroughly. Transfer to a dropper bottle, label and dispense. Attach the secondary label "For external use only.".

Uses

Sodium bicarbonate ear drops are used to relieve itching in the ears.

Marketed Ear Drops

1. Chloramphenicol ear drops (Bombay Drug House Pvt. Ltd., Bombay - 400101).

    Each ml contains:
    Chloramphenicol   5%

2. Chloromycetin ear drops [Parke-Davis (India) Ltd., Bombay - 400025].

    Contains:
    Chloramphenicol   5%
    Benzocaine 1% in propylene glycol.

3. Dexacort-N eye/ear drops (Klar Sehen Pvt. Ltd., Calcutta - 700026).

    Contains:
    Neomycin sulphate   0.5%
    Dexamethasone sod. phosphate   0.1%

4. O-Carb ear drops (Optho Remedies Pvt. Ltd., Allahabad - 211004).

    Each ml contains:
    Sod. bicarb.   34   mg
    Phenol   0.0034 ml
    Glycerin   0.34 ml

5. Ophthal eye/ear drops (Ophthal Remedies, Ahmedabad - 382455).
   Each ml contains:

Boric acid	2%
Sod. borate	0.5%
Zinc sulphate	0.1%
Glycerin	2%

Inhalations

Inhalations are the liquid preparations containing volatile ingredients and are meant for local or systemic action on the nasal or respiratory tract. If the ingredients are volatile at room temperature, they may be placed on an absorbent pad and inhaled therefrom. In other cases, they may be added to warm water, but not boiling water and the vapours are inhaled for five to ten minutes.

Inhalations are used to relieve nasal congestion and inflammation of the respiratory tract. The common examples of inhalations are benzoin inhalation, menthol and eucalyptus inhalation, ephedrine inhalation and isoproterenol hydrochloride inhalation.

Another group of products known as inhalants are drugs or combinations of drugs that can be carried into the nasal passages by virtue of their high vapour pressure. The device by which the inhalants are administered is known as inhaler. The example of an inhalant is propyl-hexedrine inhalant (Benzedrex).

Rx

Menthol	2 gm
Eucalyptus oil	10 ml
Light magnesium carbonate	7 gm
Water	up to 100 ml

Make an inhalation.

Sig: One teaspoonful to be added to 500 ml hot water (about 65°C) and inhale the vapours.

Type: Aqueous inhalation.

Procedure

Dissolve the menthol in the eucalyptus oil, add the light magnesium carbonate and sufficient water to produce 100 ml. Stir well so as to get a homogenous product. Transfer to a container, label with directions "For external use only." and "Shake the bottle before use." and dispense.

Uses

It is used as an inhalation to remove congestion of the nostrils.

Light magnesium carbonate acts as a distributing agent to ensure uniform dispersion of the oil on shaking. Light magnesium carbonate does not interfere with free volatilisation of the oil when the inhalation is added to hot water for use.

Nasal Drops

Nasal drops are usually aqueous solutions intended for instillation into the nostrils by means of dropper. They are commonly used for their antiseptic, local analgesic or vasoconstrictor properties.

At one time, oily preparation containing liquid paraffin or vegetable oils as vehicle were used to prolong the action of the drug but now the use of oily vehicles in the preparation of nasal drops is discouraged because on prolonged use the oil retards the ciliary action of the nasal mucosa or drops of oil may enter the trachea and cause lipoid pneumonia. Therefore, an aqueous vehicle is considered advisable for nasal drops.

Whenever possible nasal drops should be made iso-osmotic with 0.9% sodium chloride, pH neutral and viscosity similar to nasal secretions which can be achieved by the addition of a thickening agent like 0.5% methyl cellulose. They should be dispensed in coloured fluted bottles attached with a dropper.

Marketed Nasal Drops

1. Betnisol-N nasal drops (Glaxo India Ltd., Bombay - 400025).
   Contains:
   Betamethasone sodium phosphate 0.05%
   Naphazoline nitrate   0.05%
   Neomycin sulphate   0.5%
2. Decon nasal drops (Cadila Labs Ltd., Ahmedabad - 380050).
   Each ml contains:
   Xylometazoline HCl   0.1%
3. Diconal nasal drops (Klar Sehen Pvt. Ltd., Calcutta - 700026).
   Contains:
   Xylometazoline HCl   0.1%
   Sodium chloride   0.9%
   Glycerin   6.0%
4. Dristan nasal drops (Geoffrey Manners & Co. Ltd., Bombay - 400038).

5. Fenox nasal drops (Boots Pharmaceuticals Ltd., Bombay - 400038).
   Contains:

Phenylephrine HCl	0.25%
Naphazoline nitrate	0.025%
Chlorbutol	0.35%

6. Otrivin drops (Hindustan Ciba-Geigy Ltd., Pharmaceuticals Division, Bombay - 400020).
   Contains:

Xylometazoline HCl	0.1%

Marketed Sprays

1. Fintal nasal spray (Rallis India Ltd., Bombay - 400001).
   Contains:

Sod. cromoglycate	2% w/v
Benzalkonium chloride	0.01% w/v

2. Healex spray (Rallis India Ltd., Bombay - 400001).
   Each ml contains:

Polyvinyl polymer	2.52%
Benzocaine	0.36%
Propellant	70.0%

3. Arjet spray (Cadila Chemicals Ltd., Ahmedabad - 380050).
4. Beclate nasal spray (Cipla Ltd., Bombay - 400008).
   Each metered inhalation supplies:

Beclomethasone dipropionate	50 mcg

5. Iodex pain spray (Eskayef Ltd., Bangalore - 560049).
6. Iodex burn spray (Eskayef Ltd., Bangalore - 560049).
7. Iodex antiseptic spray (Eskayef Ltd., Bangalore - 560049).
   Contains: Povidone iodine.

2. LIQUIDS TO BE APPLIED TO THE SKIN

Liniments

Liniments are liquid or semi-liquid preparations meant for external application to the skin. They contain substances possessing analgesic, rubefacient, smoothing or stimulating properties. Liniments are usually applied to the skin with friction and rubbing of the skin. They should not be applied to the broken skin. Liniments should be dispensed in coloured fluted bottles in order to distinguish from preparations meant for internal use.

The bottle should be labelled "For external use only.".

Examples are methyl salicylate liniment, turpentine liniment, white liniment.

Storage: Liniments should be stored in tightly closed containers. The containers must bear a label "For external use only." and "Shake the bottle well before use.".

Rx

Soft soap	3.75 gm
Camphor	2.50 gm
Turpentine oil	32.50 ml
Purified water	11.25 ml

Make: Liniment.

Direction: To be applied externally to the affected part with friction.

Type: Emulsion type liniment made with an alkali soap.

Procedure

Dissolve the camphor in turpentine oil in a dry container. Separately dissolve soft soap in small amount of purified water in a mortar. To this gradually add the camphor solution with thorough trituration after each addition until a thick creamy emulsion is formed. Add sufficient purified water to produce the required volume. Transfer the preparation to a bottle, label and dispense. Apply the secondary label "For external use only." and "Shake the bottle before use.".

Uses

It acts as an irritant, counter-irritant and rubefacient.

Liniment of turpentine is applied externally to the patients suffering from arthralgia (pain in the joints), myalgia (muscular pain), fibrositis (ligamental pain) and sprain.

1. Irritants are the agents or substances which do not directly destroy the tissues but cause inflammation in the area to which they are applied.
2. Rubefacients are the substances which produce congestion and redness of the area to which they are applied, producing the initial symptoms of irritation.
3. Counter-irritants are the agents or drugs which are applied locally to irritate the intact skin thus reducing or relieving another irritation or deep seated pain. They seem to work by producing an

inflammation, thus increasing the flow of blood to the affected area. Physical counter-irritants include hot water bottles, radiant heat, short wave diathermy and galvanic electric current. Chemical counterirritants include volatile substances like turpentine oil, camphor, menthol, thymol and methyl salicylate.

4. Since turpentine oil is a volatile oil which is not miscible with water, to make them miscible with each other soft soap has been used which acts as an emulsifying agent.

5. Turpentine oil is a volatile oil obtained by the distillation and rectification of turpentine which is an oleoresin obtained from various species of pinus.

6. Camphor is a volatile substance obtained from wood of cinnamomum camphora. It can be prepared synthetically. Externally it acts as a mild analgesic and rubefacient. It is used as a counter-irritant in the treatment of fibrositis and neuralgia.

Precautions

Liniments are not to be applied to the broken skin because they may produce excessive irritation of the skin.

Marketed Liniments

1. Turpentine liniment (Alpine Industries, New Delhi - 110028).
   Each contains:

Soft soap	90 gm
Camphor	50 gm
Turpentine oil	650 ml
Purified water to	1000 ml

2. Turpentine liniment (Agrawal Pharmaceuticals, Delhi - 110092).
3. Turpentine liniment (Arora Pharmaceuticals, Delhi - 110035).
4. Methyl salicylate liniment (Alpine Industries, New Delhi - 110028).
   Each contains:

Methyl salicylate	250 mg
Arachis oil to	1000 ml

Marketed Applications

1. Ascazol application (Indian National Drug Co. Pvt. Ltd., Calcutta - 700085).
   Contains:

Benzyl benzoate	25%

2. Benzyl benzoate application (Medo Chem Lab. Pvt. Ltd., Delhi - 110032).
   Each contains:

Benzyl benzoate	250 gm
Emulsifying wax	20 gm
Purified water to	1000 ml

3. Benzyl benzoate application (Agrawal Pharmaceuticals, Delhi - 110092).
4. Benzyl benzoate application (Rays Labs. Pvt. Ltd., Calcutta - 700007).

Lotions

Lotions are usually suspensions or dispersions intended for external application to the skin. They are applied directly to the skin without rubbing with the help of some absorbent material such as cotton wool or the cotton wool or gauze soaked in the lotion is applied to the affected part. Lotions may be employed for local cooling, soothing or protective purposes. Dermatologists frequently prescribe lotions for anaesthetic or antiseptic actions. The inclusion of alcohol in a lotion hastens its drying and produces cooling effect whereas the addition of glycerin in a lotion keeps the skin moist for sufficiently long time and does not allow the preparation to dry.

Bacteria and molds grow in certain lotions if no preservative is added to the preparation. Even if a preservative is added care must be taken to avoid contamination during preparation of the lotion.

Lotions should be dispensed in coloured fluted bottles in order to distinguish from preparations meant for internal use. The container should be labelled "For external use only.". On long standing the lotions have a tendency to separate out. Therefore, the container must be labelled "Shake before use.".

Examples are calamine lotion, oily calamine lotion, salicylic acid lotion and zinc sulphate lotion.

Lotions Containing Insoluble Substances

When a lotion contains insoluble substances of indiffusible nature, it will have to be dispensed in lotions like that of mixtures, i.e., by incorporating a suspending agent. For this purpose gummy suspending agents like tragacanth is not suitable because of their sticky nature. Therefore, bentonite and aluminium hydroxide gel are sometimes used as suspending agents.

Calamine lotion is the best example of lotions containing insoluble substances. This lotion contains calamine, zinc oxide, bentonite, sodium citrate, liquefied phenol, glycerin and purified water.

Here calamine is an insoluble substance of indiffusible nature. It acts as astringent, soothing and protective agent. Zinc oxide is an adjuvant, it acts as mild astringent with local soothing, protective and antiseptic properties. Bentonite acts as a suspending agent which swells up in water and imparts viscosity to the solution. Sodium citrate is incorporated to prevent the lotion from being too viscous. Liquefied phenol is used as an antiseptic and glycerin as a humectant.

Method of Preparation

Triturate calamine, zinc oxide and bentonite with a portion of sodium citrate solution in a mortar till a smooth cream is formed. Add remaining amount of sodium citrate solution and mix well. Incorporate glycerin and liquefied phenol, mix thoroughly. Add more of vehicle to produce the required volume. Stir thoroughly so as to get a homogeneous product.

Rx

Calamine	15.0 gm
Zinc oxide	5.0 gm
Bentonite	3.0 gm
Sodium citrate	0.5 gm
Liquefied phenol	0.5 ml
Glycerin	5.0 ml
Purified water up to	100.0 ml

Make: Lotion. Send 50 ml.

Direction: To be applied to the affected part of the skin without friction.

Procedure

Mix the weighed amount of calamine, zinc oxide and bentonite in a mortar. Triturate it with a solution of sodium citrate in about 70 ml of purified water. Add the required quantity of liquefied phenol and glycerin. Mix well. To this add more of vehicle to produce the required volume. Mix thoroughly so as to get a uniform preparation. Transfer to a bottle, cork, label and dispense. Apply the secondary label "Shake the bottle before use." and "For external use only.".

Uses

This lotion is used as an astringent and protectant from sunburn. It acts as a soothening agent and gives relief from itching and pain during skin irritation. It is also used in ringworm infection and eczema.

1. Calamine is basic zinc carbonate mixed with suitable amount of ferric oxide to impart pink colour. It is often prescribed by dermatologists to give flesh like colour to lotions or creams.

2. Zinc oxide has mild astringent, protective and antiseptic action. It is widely used in dusting powders, lotion, and ointments meant for the treatment of skin diseases and infections such as eczema, ringworm, psoriasis (chronic skin disease in which red scaly patches develop) and pruritus (itching).

3. Bentonite is a native colloidal hydrated aluminium silicate. It is insoluble in water but swells up nearly seven times its bulk and forms a magma with desirable viscosity. Hence it is used as suspending agent for the dispersion of insoluble substances like calamine, etc.

4. Sodium citrate is added to prevent the lotion from being too viscous. It acts as a buffer and maintains the pH appropriate for skin preparations.

5. Liquefied phenol acts as antipruritic because of its antiseptic properties and also because of its local anaesthetic action.

6. Glycerin acts as a hygroscopic thus keeps the skin moist and have soothening effect on the skin.

Marketed Lotions

1. Caladryl lotion [Parke-Davis (India) Ltd., Bombay - 400025].
   Contains:

Calamine	8% w/v
Camphor	0.1% w/v
Diphenhydramine HCl	1% w/v
Special denatured spirit	2.37% v/v

2. Calderm skin lotion (Dermocare Labs, Ahmedabad - 380001).
   Contains:

Calamine	15% w/w

Zinc oxide	5% w/w
Glycerin	5% w/w

3. Calamine lotion (Alpine Industries, New Delhi - 110028).
   Each contains:

Calamine	160 gm
Zinc oxide	50 gm
Bentonite	30 gm
Sod. citrate	5 gm
Liquefied phenol	5 ml
Glycerin	50 ml
Rose water	1000 ml

4. Calamine lotion [Jilichem Labs (India) Ltd., Ahmedabad - 382445].
5. Calamine lotion (Agrawal Pharmaceuticals, Delhi - 110092).
6. Senee hair lotion (Dermocare Labs, Ahmedabad - 380001).

SUSPENSIONS

Suspensions are the biphasic liquid dosage form of medicament in which the finely divided solid particles ranging from 0.5 to 5.0 micron are suspended or dispersed in a liquid or semi-solid vehicle. The solid particles constitutes the discontinuous phase whereas the liquid vehicle constitutes the continuous phase. Suspensions are mainly used for oral administration, external application or parenteral use. Oral suspensions can be made more palatable by using derivative of the drug as in the case of chloramphenicol palmitate. Suspensions are also chemically more stable than solutions. That is why now a days many suspensions are marketed as dry powders and the patient or pharmacist is asked to incorporate a specified amount of the vehicle to constitute the suspension before its use. Suspension is an ideal dosage form for patients who cannot swallow tablets or capsules. Suspensions meant for external application should have very small particle size to avoid gritty feeling to the skin. Similarly suspensions meant for introduction into the ophthalmic cavity should be free from gritty particles to avoid irritation, pain and discomfort. In some cases, sterile suspensions are injected hypodermically to produce sustained action of the drug which will not be produced by a true solution of the same drug.

Qualities of Good Suspension

A well formulated suspension should have the following properties:

1. The dispersed particles should not settle readily and the settled particles should redisperse immediately on shaking.
2. The particles should not form a cake on settling.
3. The viscosity should be such that the preparation can be easily poured.
4. It should be chemically stable.
5. Suspensions for internal use must be palatable and suspensions for external use must be free from gritty particles and possess other characteristics required for external preparations.

Flocculated and Non-Flocculated Suspensions

In flocculated suspensions the individual particles are in contact with each other to form loose aggregates and create a network like structure. Although the rate of sedimentation is high but the sediment is loosely packed which can redisperse easily on shaking so as to reform the original suspension. However the flocculated suspensions meant for oral, parenteral, ophthalmic or external use may not be elegant because they are difficult to remove from bottles or vials and on transferring from the bottle the floccules remain sticking to the sides of the bottle. These properties can be improved by adding protective colloids.

In non-flocculated or de-flocculated suspensions all individual particles exist as separate entities. The rate of sedimentation is slow and a sediment is formed slowly but the sediment is closely packed due to weight of upper layers of sedimenting materials. A hard cake is formed which is difficult to redisperse to get original suspension. The non-flocculated suspensions have pleasing appearance as compared to flocculated suspensions because the substances remain suspended for a sufficiently long time.

Formulation of Suspensions

Before selecting the additives to be used in the formulation of suspensions it is very important to decide whether the particles in suspension are to be flocculated or to remain non-flocculated. Following are the additives which are generally used in the formulation of suspensions:
1. Flocculating agents
2. Suspending agents/thickening agents
3. Wetting agents
4. Dispersing agents

Relative Properties of Flocculated and Non-Flocculated Suspensions

Flocculated	*Non-Flocculated*
1. Particles form loose aggregates and form a network-like structure.	Particles exist as separate entities.
2. Rate of sedimentation is high.	Rate of sedimentation is slow.
3. Sediment is rapidly formed.	Sediment is slowly formed.
4. Sediment is loosely packed and does not form a hard cake.	Sediment is very closely packed and a hard cake is formed.
5. Sediment is easy to redisperse.	Sediment is difficult to redisperse.
6. Suspension is not pleasing in appearance.	Suspension is pleasing in appearance.
7. The floccules stick to the sides of the bottle.	They do not stick to the sides of the bottle.

5. Preservative
6. Organoleptic additives.

1. Flocculating Agents

When formulating suspensions it must be ensured that the particles are well dispersed in the vehicle. The dispersion can be improved by adding a surfactant which will act by reducing the interfacial tension. For example, if surfactants with negative charges are adsorbed on the particles, prevents or minimises flocculation in the presence of positive ions because of natural repulsion of like charges. Sodium lauryl sulphate and sodium dioctyl sulphosuccinate are examples of this type of surfactants. Non-ionic surfactants also usually assume a negative charge in solution thereby act as effective flocculating agents. Generally non-ionic surfactants are used for dispersing the insoluble particles. Tweens, spans and carbowaxes are frequently used in this manner.

Protective colloids can also be used as flocculating agents. They differ from surfactants in that they do not reduce the interfacial tension. Their solutions differ in viscosity and are used in higher concentration than surfactants.

2. Suspending Agents/Thickening Agents

Suspending agents are the substances which are added to a suspension to increase the viscosity of the continuous phase so that the particles remain suspended for a sufficiently long time and it becomes easy to measure an accurate dose.

While selecting a suspending agent it is not only important that it should increase the viscosity of the system but the pourability, spreadability, etc., of the final product must also be taken into consideration. Some of the thickening agents used in formulations include acacia, tragacanth and sodium alginate. As these are natural products therefore vary in qualities and properties hence not very commonly used. The semi-synthetic thickening agents widely used include methyl cellulose, carboxy methyl cellulose, hydroxypropyl methyl cellulose, synthetic polymers and gelatin. Sodium carboxy methyl cellulose in concentration of about 3.5% is used in injectable suspensions. Clays such as hydrated aluminium silicate or magnesium silicate are also used as suspending agents. Non-ionic substances such as sorbitol, glycerin, sugar or polyethylene glycols may be included to adjust the viscosity of the medium.

3. Wetting Agents

Wetting agents are the substances which reduce the interfacial tension between the solid particles and liquid medium thus producing a suspension of desired quality. This may be achieved by adding a suitable wetting agent which is adsorbed at the solid/liquid interface in such a way that the affinity of the particles for the surrounding medium is increased and the interparticular forces are decreased. Examples of wetting agents are alcohol in tragacanth mucilage, glycerin and glycols in sodium alginate or bentonite dispersions and polysorbates in oral and parenteral suspensions.

Only a minimum amount of wetting agent should be used; excessive amounts may lead to foaming or impart an undesirable taste or odour to the suspension.

4. Dispersing Agents

The first step in the formulation of any suspension is to ensure that the particles are dispersed in and wetted by the dispersion medium. In some substances where the surface energy is not sufficient the particles may come together and form larger particles. To overcome this difficulty the substances which are used are known as dispersing agents. They carry good charge and are easily adsorbed on to the disperse phase particles. These substances increase the zeta potential and do not allow the particles to come together to form large particles.

5. Preservative

The presence of suspending agents and medicaments which are liable for bacterial growth makes it necessary to incorporate a preservative in suspensions. Preservatives selected should be effective against a wide range of micro-organisms and should be chemically and physically stable. It should be non-toxic and compatible with other added substances. The commonly used preservatives are benzoic acid, sodium benzoate, methyl paraben and propyl-paraben.

6. Organoleptic Additives

Colours, sweetening agents and flavouring agents are used in oral suspensions. Similarly colours and perfumes are incorporated in suspensions meant for external application but these must be compatible with other ingredients.

Preparation of Suspensions

These preparations are generally of two types:
1. Those in which the insoluble substances are added to the vehicle or the vehicle is added to the insoluble substances.
2. Those in which the insoluble material is formed in the liquid due to the interaction of two or more ingredients.

Some of the preparations can be made by both of these methods, others by only one method but most of the preparations containing insoluble materials are prepared by the first method, i.e., by adding the insoluble material to the vehicle.

(a) Suspensions Containing Diffusible Solids

Diffusible solids are those substances which do not dissolve in water, but on shaking they can be mixed with it and remain evenly distributed through- out the liquid for sufficiently long time allowing uniform distribution of the drug in each dose. However, on standing, the insoluble solids settle at the bottom of the bottle which require re-shaking of the bottle each time whenever a dose is to be measured. Hence the bottle containing the diffusible mixture must be labelled "Shake the bottle before use.". Diffusible solids include aromatic chalk powder, bismuth carbonate, light kaolin, magnesium oxide, light magnesium carbonate, heavy magnesium carbonate, magnesium trisilicate, phenolphthalein, rhubarb powder.

Method of Dispensing

Finely powder the diffusible and other substances (if they are already not in fine powder) in a mortar. Mix them thoroughly. Add a small amount of vehicle out of 3/4 th measured out vehicle and triturate to make a smooth cream. (Due to the presence of air in the interstices of many powders, they float at the surface of water and do not mix with the vehicle. To prevent this tendency, a smooth cream is prepared by adding a small amount of vehicle at first and then diluted.) Add the remainder of vehicle. If foreign particles are visible pass the suspension through a piece of muslin but if one or two foreign particles are visible, remove them with a glass rod. Add liquid ingredients and make up the required volume by adding more of vehicle. Transfer the suspension to a bottle, cork, polish, label and dispense. "Shake the bottle before use." label must be attached.

Rx

Light kaolin	2.0 gm
Light magnesium carbonate	0.5 gm
Sodium bicarbonate	0.5 gm
Peppermint water q.s.	15.0 ml

Make a mixture. Send six doses.
Direction: One dose to be taken three times a day.
Type: Mixture containing diffusible solids.

(b) Suspensions Containing Indiffusible Solids

Indiffusible solids are those substances which do not dissolve in water and do not remain evenly distributed in the vehicle for sufficiently long time to ensure uniformity of the measured dose. This difficulty is overcome by increasing the viscosity of the vehicle for which purpose suspending agents are used. The two commonly used suspending agents are (a) compound tragacanth powder which is used in the ratio of 2 gm per 100 ml of the suspension or 10 grain per ounce of the suspension to be prepared (b) tragacanth mucilage, it is used in the ratio of 1/4 th of the volume of the suspension to be prepared. Tragacanth mucilage is used only when the vehicle is chloroform water or water because mucilage is prepared by using chloroform water and if added to preparations containing medicinally active vehicle may replace some of the medicinally active vehicle thereby decreasing their activity. In such cases compound tragacanth powder must be used as suspending agent. Indiffusible solids include: for oral suspensions — aspirin, aromatic chalk powder, phenobarbitone, succinyl sulphathiazole, sulphadimidine; and for externally used suspensions — calamine, sulphur precipitated, zinc oxide.

For its preparation, finely powder the indiffusible substance in a mortar, add any soluble or diffusible solids and compound tragacanth powder or tragacanth mucilage and mix thoroughly. If only indiffusible substance is to be incorporated, mix it with compound tragacanth powder in a mortar. Add sufficient amount of vehicle and triturate so as to form a smooth cream. Then add more of vehicle to form a pourable liquid. Remove the foreign particles and proceed further as described under suspensions containing diffusible solids.

Rx

Succinyl sulphathiazole, in powder	1.0 gm
Light kaolin	0.6 gm
Compound tragacanth powder	0.1 gm
Raspberry syrup	2.0 ml
Benzoic acid solution	0.2 ml
Amaranth solution	0.1 ml
Chloroform water to produce	10.0 ml

Fiat mistura. Mitte 90 ml.
Signa: Cochleare amplum ter in die sumenda.
Type: Mixture containing indiffusible solids.

(c) Suspensions Produced by Chemical Reactions

In this type of preparation of suspensions the highly diluted solutions of the reacting substances are mixed together so as to form very finely divided precipitates that can be easily distributed throughout the liquid by shaking. Precipitates so formed are generally diffusible in nature therefore there is no need of adding any suspending agent. Zinc sulphide lotion B.P.C. is prepared in this way.

Suspensions Containing Precipitate-forming Liquids

Precipitate forming liquids include: compound benzoin tincture, benzoin tincture, lobelia ethereal tincture, myrrh tincture, tolu tincture. These liquids are not only insoluble in water but they form indiffusible precipitates particularly when salts are present. They contain resinous matter and when mixed with water lead to precipitation of the resin and may stick to the sides of the bottle which will be difficult to rediffuse by shaking. To prevent this tendency a suspending agent like compound tragacanth powder 2 gm/100 ml or tragacanth mucilage 1/4 th of the total volume to be prepared, will have to be incorporated.

1. Method of preparation using compound traganth powder

This method is very convenient when diffusible or indiffusible solids are also included in the prescription and must be used when the vehicle is water or medicinally active.

Finely powder any insoluble solid if already not in powder form and mix it with compound tragacanth powder in a mortar (If no solid ingredient is to be used then place the compound tragacanth powder alone in the mortar.) Measure out half of the vehicle and incorporate a small amount out of it to the powders with thorough trituration until a smooth cream is formed. Then add the remainder amount of the vehicle.

Measure the precipitate forming liquid in a dry measure and add it in a slow stream in the centre of the cream with rapid stirring. Pouring the sticky liquid on the pestle or the sides of the mortar must be avoided.

Dissolve the soluble ingredient (if present) in sufficient amount of vehicle out of remaining half of the vehicle. Add it slowly with constant stirring to the cream to avoid local high concentrations that might neutralize the effect of suspending agent.

Examine the contents of the mortar critically. If foreign particles are visible pass the suspension through a piece of muslin but if one or two foreign particles are visible remove them with a glass rod. Add more of vehicle to produce the final volume. Transfer the suspension to a bottle, cork, polish, label and dispense. "Shake the bottle before use." label must be attached.

2. Method of preparation using tragacanth mucilage

This method is more rapid than the first method and may be used when insoluble solids are absent and the vehicle used is water or chloroform water.

Mix the tragacanth mucilage with an equal volume of vehicle. Measure the precipitate-forming liquid in a dry measure and pour in the centre of the mucilage with constant stirring.

Dissolve any soluble substances in 1/4 th of the vehicle and add to the above mixture. Examine the contents critically and remove any foreign particles. Transfer the suspension to a bottle, cork, polish, label and dispense. "Shake the bottle before use." label must be attached.

Rx

Potassium iodide	4 gm
Lobelia ethereal tincture	16 ml
Stramonium tincture	32 ml
Chloroform water q.s.	180 ml

Fiat mistura.

Signa: Cochleare magnum quarter in die sumenda.

Type: Mixture containing precipitate forming liquid.

Theory

Lobelia ethereal tincture is a precipitate forming liquid so a suspending agent will have to be added. The vehicle is chloroform water and there are no insoluble substances present. Therefore follow the method for precipitate forming liquids using tragacanth mucilage as suspending agent. Potassium iodide must be added after dilution and with continuous stirring.

Packaging and Storage

Oral suspensions should be packaged in wide mouth containers so that they can be easily removed from them and without any delay. All the containers in which suspensions are filled should have sufficient space above the liquid to permit adequate shaking. They must be labelled "Shake well." and it must be ensured to shake the bottle each time when taking the dose so as to evenly distribute the particles throughout the vehicle.

Physical stability of suspensions is greatly affected by extremes of temperatures. Suspensions should be stored in a cool place but should not be kept in refrigerator which may damage the product. Freezing should be avoided which may lead to aggregation of the suspended particles.

Marketed Suspensions

1. Acemiz suspension (Lupin Laboratories Ltd., Bombay - 400098).

    Each 5 ml contains:
    Astemizole   5 mg

2. Bactrim suspension (Roche Products Ltd., Bombay - 400034).

    Each 5 ml contains:
    Trimethoprim   40 mg
    Sulphamethoxazole   200 mg

3. Chloramphenicol palmitate suspension (Klar Sehen Pvt. Ltd., Calcutta - 700026).

    Each 5 ml contains:
    Chloramphenicol palmitate eq. to Chloramphenicol 125 mg

4. Dependal-M suspension (Eskayef Limited, Bangalore - 560049).

    Each 5 ml contains:
    Furazolidone   25 mg
    Metronidazole   75 mg

5. Campicillin (paediatric) suspension (Cadila Laboratories Ltd., Ahmedabad - 380050).

    Each ml contains:
    Ampicillin anhydrous   100 mg

6. Penetrin suspension (Cyanamid India Ltd., Lederle Division, Bombay - 400025).

    Each 5 ml contains:
    Trimethoprim   40 mg
    Sulphadimidine   200 mg

7. Septran suspension (Burroughs Wellcome India Ltd., Bombay - 400023).

    Each 5 ml contains:
    Trimethoprim   40 mg
    Sulphamethonazole   200 mg

8. Wormin suspension (Cadila Laboratories Ltd., Ahmedabad - 380050).

    Each 5 ml contains:
    Mebendazole   100 mg

EMULSIONS

An emulsion is a liquid preparation containing two immiscible liquids, one of which is dispersed as minute globules into the other. The liquid that is broken up into globules is called the dispersed phase or internal phase and the liquid in which the globules are dispersed is known as continuous or external phase. The globules remain dispersed only for a short time and separation takes place quickly upon standing. Therefore a third substance known as emulsifying agent is added to the system which forms a film around the globules of the dispersed phase thereby the globules remain scattered indefinitely in the continuous phase and a uniform, stable product is formed.

An emulsion may also be defined as a biphasic liquid dosage form of medicament in which two immiscible liquids (generally one of which is water and the other is some lipid or oil) are made miscible by the addition of a third substance known as emulgent or emulsifying agent.

Emulsions are widely used in pharmacy and medicine. They are used internally as well as externally. Certain medicinal agents having an unpleasant taste and odour can be made more palatable for oral administration in the form of emulsions, which are otherwise difficult to take, e.g., cod-liver oil, castor oil, etc. The activity of certain drugs can be increased and action can be prolonged by emulsifying the drug in a suitable vehicle. Sterile stable intravenous emulsions containing fats, carbohydrates and vitamins all in one preparation can be administered to the patients who are unable to take these vital substances by oral route. Dermatological preparations like creams and lotions are extensively formulated as emulsions. Most recently the foam aerosols have been developed in the form of emulsions.

Types of Emulsions

There are two types of emulsions:
(a) Oil in water type (O/W)
(b) Water in oil type (W/O).

In oil in water type emulsions the oil is in the dispersed phase whereas water is in the continuous phase. These types of emulsions are prepared by using emulsifying agents like gum acacia, tragacanth, methyl cellulose, saponins, synthetic substances and soaps formed from monovalent bases like Na^+, K^+ and NH_4^+. Oil in water type emulsions are preferred for internal use because the unpleasant taste and odour is masked by emulsification and oil being in a finely dispersed state is more quickly assimilated in the body.

In water in oil type emulsions, the water is in the dispersed phase whereas oil is in the continuous phase. These types of emulsions are mainly used externally as lotions or creams. Some oil in water type emulsions can also be used externally. The type of emulsifying agent used will determine the kind of emulsion formed. Antiseptics and other medicaments are more effective when used in the form of oil in water type emulsions. When an emollient action is required then water in oil emulsions are used externally. Emulsifying agents like wool fat, resins, bees wax, synthetic compounds and soaps formed from divalent bases like Ca^{++}, Mg^{++} and Zn^{++} are used for the preparation of water in oil emulsions.

Microemulsions

Clear dispersions of oil in water or water in oil are referred to as micro-emulsions. These appear homogeneous to the naked eye. These types of emulsions are also known as solubilized systems because macroscopically they seem to behave as true solutions but these micro-emulsions should not be confused with solutions formed by co-solvency.

Microemulsions can be prepared with emulsifying agents which give a local negative interfacial tension and form monomolecular interfacial films. Since these are clear preparations so becoming more popular day by day. Microemulsions are also free from some of the stability problems of emulsions.

Tests for Identification of Type of Emulsion

Since both the types (O/W) and (W/O) of emulsions are similar in appearance therefore it is very difficult to differentiate them with naked eye. They can be identified with the help of following tests but no one test gives correct results. Therefore the type of emulsion determined by one method should be confirmed by second method.

(a) Dilution Test

Take a few drops of emulsion in a test-tube and dilute it with 2-3 drops of water. If the water is distributed uniformly in the emulsion then the emulsion is O/W type but if water separates out as a layer then the emulsion is W/O type. Similarly on dilution with oil, the oil will distribute uniformly in W/O emulsion but separates out in O/W type emulsion.

(b) Conductivity Test

Water is a good conductor of electricity whereas oil is non-conductor of electricity. So conductivity test can be performed by dipping a pair of electrodes connected through a low voltage lamp, in the emulsion. On passing an electric current through the electrodes if the bulb glows, the emulsion is O/W type because water is in the continuous phase and current has passed through the water but if the bulb does not glow, the emulsion is W/O type because oil is in the continuous phase and the current has not passed through the oil which has failed to glow the bulb.

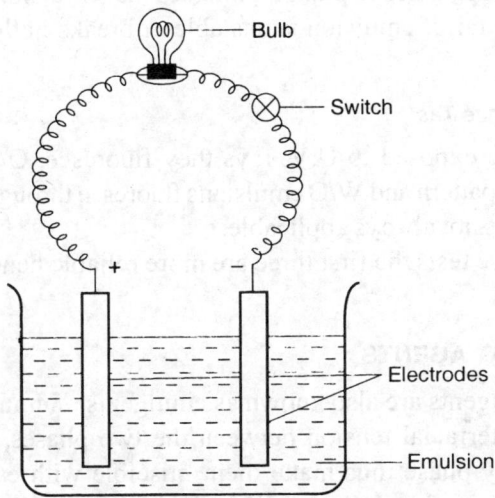

Fig. 10.4. Conductivity test.

(c) Dye-Solubility Test

Mix an oil soluble dye like scarlet red with an emulsion. Place a drop of it on a microscope slide and see under the microscope. If the continuous phase appears to be red, it is W/O emulsion but if scattered globules appears red and continuous phase colourless it is O/W emulsion. This test can be repeated by using amaranth, a water soluble dye. If the continuous phase appears red it is O/W emulsion but if scattered globules appear red and continuous phase colourless it is W/O emulsion.

(d) CoCl₂ Filter Paper Test

When a filter paper impregnated with $CoCl_2$ and dried (blue) is dipped

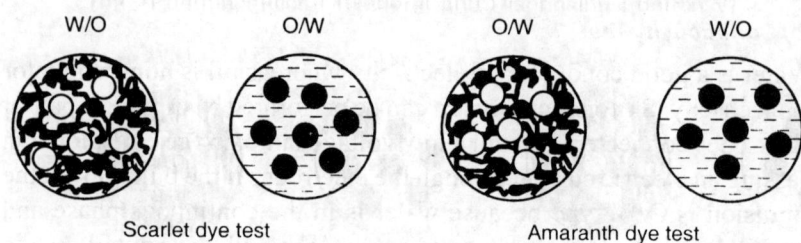

Fig. 10.5. Dye-solubility test.

in an emulsion changes to pink, it indicates that emulsion is O/W type. This test may fail if emulsion is unstable or breaks in the presence of electrolytes.

(e) Fluorescence Test

When oils are exposed to U.V. rays they fluoresce, O/W emulsions exhibit spotty pattern and W/O emulsions fluoresce throughout the field. This method is not always applicable.

Out of these tests the first three are more reliable hence commonly used.

EMULSIFYING AGENTS

Emulsifying agents are also known as emulgents of emulsifiers. They reduce the interfacial tension between the two phases, i.e., aqueous phase and oily phase thus make them miscible with each other and form a stable emulsion. It is very difficult to select a proper emulsifying agent for the development of a stable emulsion.

No single emulsifying agent possesses all the properties required for the preparation of stable emulsion therefore sometimes it becomes necessary to use two or more than two emulsifying agents instead of one to get a product of desired qualities.

Classification of Emulsifying Agents

Emulsifying agents may be classified as follows:

1. Natural emulsifying agents from vegetable sources
    (a) Acacia
    (b) Tragacanth
    (c) Agar
    (d) Chondrus (Irish Moss)

(e) Pectin

(f) Starch.

2. Natural emulsifying agents from animal sources
   (a) Gelatin
   (b) Egg yolk
   (c) Wool fat.

3. Semi-synthetic polysaccharides
   (a) Methyl cellulose
   (b) Sodium carboxymethyl cellulose.

4. Synthetic emulsifying agents
   (a) Anionic
   (b) Cationic
   (c) Non-ionic.

5. Inorganic emulsifying agents
   (a) Milk of magnesia
   (b) Magnesium oxide
   (c) Magnesium trisilicate
   (d) Magnesium aluminium silicate
   (e) Bentonite

6. Saponins

7. Alcohols
   (a) Cholesterol
   (b) Carbowaxes
   (c) Lecithin.

1. Natural Emulsifying Agents from Vegetable Sources

The natural emulsifying agents obtained from vegetable sources are carbohydrates which include gums and mucilaginous substances. They are anionic in nature and produce O/W emulsions. Some of them act as true emulsifiers which are also known as primary emulsifying agents while others act as emulsion stabilizers also known as secondary emulsifying agents. They are capable of emulsifying a large number of substances but the resulting emulsions will have to be preserved by adding a suitable preservative because the carbohydrates act as very good medium for bacterial growth. The preservatives which can be added are alcohol, sodium benzoate, benzoic acid or a combination of methyl paraben and propyl paraben. These preservatives should be added carefully because high concentrations of alcohols and solutions of metallic salts may lead to cracking of emulsion.

(a) Acacia

Acacia is the best known emulsifying agent for the extemporaneous preparation of emulsions for internal use. Emulsions prepared with gum acacia are attractive in appearance, quite palatable and relatively stable. They are stable over a wide range of pH (2 to 10). These emulsions usually have low viscosity therefore creaming takes place quite rapidly which can be prevented by increasing the viscosity of the medium by incorporating tragacanth, agar or pectin along with acacia.

Emulsions prepared with acacia are susceptible to bacterial growth therefore they must be suitably preserved.

The ratio of powdered acacia usually taken for emulsification of fixed oils is 1: 4 and for volatile oils is 1: 2, that is 1 gram of acacia is sufficient to emulsify 4 ml of fixed oils and 2 ml of volatile oils. When mucilage of acacia is used, 1 gram is sufficient for 2 ml of oil.

(b) Tragacanth

Tragacanth alone is rarely used as an emulsifying agent because it does not reduce the interfacial tension and thus the oil globules are usually of large size. It produces very coarse and thick emulsions and sometimes viscosity increases to such an extent that pouring of the emulsion becomes a problem. A very stable emulsion is produced if both acacia and tragacanth are used as emulsifying agents for the preparation of an emulsion. Tragacanth will render the emulsion more viscous and thereby the rate of creaming will be reduced which is quite high in the case of acacia emulsions. The quantity of tragacanth required for this purpose is 1/10 th of the amount of acacia used. The appearance and stability of the emulsions can be improved to a great extent by passing the finished product through a homogenizer.

(c) Agar

Agar is not a good emulsifying agent as it forms a very coarse and viscous emulsion. It is commonly used as a thickening agent along with acacia for the emulsification of mineral oils. Generally 2% mucilage of agar is prepared by dissolving it in boiling water and cooled to 45°C. Below this temperature it will form a gel which is not used in emulsions.

The mucilage is incorporated in the primary emulsion in sufficient quantity to make 30 to 50 per cent of the final volume.

(d) Chondrus (Irish Moss)

Like agar, chondrus is also not used as a primary emulsifier but is used as a thickening agent. Generally it is used along with acacia for the emulsification of cod-liver oil and to mask the unpleasant odour and taste of the oil. A 3% solution is used to emulsify an equal volume of the oil.

(e) Pectin

Pectin is a purified complex carbohydrate obtained from the inner rind of citrus fruit and from the pulp of apple and guava. It acts as a emulsion stabilizer in acacia emulsions. If pectin alone is to be used as emulsifying agent a ratio of 0.1 gm per gram of acacia is sufficient for emulsification of the oil. A mucilage of pectin is first prepared before adding it to the preparation. To prevent the formation of lumps, pectin can be triturated with a small amount of alcohol, glycerol or syrup before the addition of water.

(f) Starch

Starch is rarely used as an emulsifying agent but the use of starch mucilage is restricted to preparations used as enemas.

2. Natural Emulsifying Agents from Animal Sources

(a) Gelatin

Gelatin is mainly used for the emulsification of liquid paraffin. 1% concentration forms the emulsions. Emulsions so formed are quite white and have an agreeable taste. However gelatin emulsions are prone to bacterial growth therefore a suitable preservative must be incorporated.

(b) Egg Yolk

Egg yolk itself is an emulsion because of the presence of lecithin and cholesterol which act as emulsifying agents. It is rarely used in industrial preparations because the emulsions are spoiled during transportation, therefore it is mainly used in extemporaneous preparations meant for internal use. It is generally used for the emulsification of fish liver oils. On an average 15 gram of egg yolk can be obtained from each egg which can emulsify about 120 ml of fixed oil and 60 ml of volatile oil. A suitable preservative must be added to emulsions prepared with egg yolk and further they must be stored in a refrigerator.

(c) Wool Fat (Anhydrous Lanolin)

Wool fat is generally used in emulsions meant for external application. It produces water in oil emulsions and can absorb about 50% of water but when mixed with other fatty substances it can emulsify several times its own weight of water and other hydroalcoholic liquids.

3. Semi-Synthetic Polysaccharides

(a) Methyl Cellulose

Methyl cellulose is a synthetic derivative of cellulose and is widely used in the pharmaceutical industry as suspending, thickening and emulsifying agent. It is available in different forms such as methyl cellulose 20, methyl cellulose 2500 and methyl cellulose 4500. The number indicates the average viscosity in centipoises of a 2 per cent aqueous solution. Methyl cellulose is commonly used for emulsification of mineral and vegetable oils but is less satisfactory for cod liver oil. Methyl cellulose is soluble in hot water therefore a special technique is used for quick preparation of mucilage. Emulsions prepared with methyl cellulose are very stable to pH changes and alcohol but may be precipitated in the presence of large amounts of electrolytes.

(b) Sodium Carboxymethyl Cellulose

It is not used as a true emulsifier but is used as an emulsion stabilizer in the concentration of 0.5 to 1.0%. It is soluble in cold water as well as hot water.

4. Synthetic Emulsifying Agents

This group includes the surface active agents which are used as emulsifying agents. They are classified according to the ionic charge possessed by the molecules of the surfactant, e.g., anionic, cationic and non-ionic.

(a) Anionic

Various alkali soaps, metallic soaps, sulphated alcohols and sulphonates are used as emulsifying agents. They bear a negative charge on them. Soaps may be used as very good emulsifying agents but are mainly meant for external application. Soap emulsions have a high pH and are not stable at pH values less than 10. They are also precipitated by the addition of acids and electrolytes.

Among the sulphated alcohols, sodium lauryl sulphate is commonly used as emulsifying agent in topical preparations. It produces O/W emulsions.

Dioctyl sodium sulphosuccinate is an example of sulphonates which is widely used in the preparations of materials which are used to soften the stools. It is also used in topical preparations.

(b) Cationic

Cationic surface active agents bear positive charge on them. They are mainly used in the preparations meant for external use such as skin lotions and creams. They have marked bacterial properties therefore generally reserved for those preparations in which germicidal activity is required.

Quaternary ammonium compounds are the only group of cationic agents which are extensively used as emulsifying agents. These include benzalkonium chloride, benzethonium chloride, cetrimide, etc.

(c) Non-Ionic

The non-ionic surface active agents are widely used in the preparation of pharmaceutical emulsions because the emulsions prepared with non-ionic surfactants remain stable over a wide range of pH changes and are not affected by the addition of acids and electrolytes. The most commonly used non-ionic surface active agents are the glyceryl esters such as glyceryl monostearate, polyoxyethylene glycol esters and ethers, and sorbitan fatty acid esters such as sorbitan monopalmitate.

5. Inorganic Emulsifying Agents

Several inorganic substances such as milk of magnesia, magnesium oxide, magnesium trisilicate, magnesium aluminium silicate, bentonite, etc., are used in the preparation of pharmaceutical emulsions. Usually they produce O/W emulsions but bentonite may be used to prepare either O/W or W/O emulsions, depending on the order of mixing. 5% suspension of bentonite is used as an emulsifying agent. For the preparation of O/W emulsion, oil is added to the suspension of bentonite whereas for W/O emulsion the oil is placed in the container and then the bentonite suspension is added to the oil with rapid stirring.

6. Saponins

Saponins are rarely used as emulsifying agents. If specially prescribed then quillaia tincture and liquid extract may be used as emulsifying agents.

7. Alcohols

(a) Cholesterol

A number of high molecular weight alcohols are used in emulsion systems primarily for their stabilizing action. Cetyl alcohol, stearyl alcohol, cholesterol and glyceryl monostearate may be included in this group. They are rarely used as single emulsifying agent therefore other emulsifying agents must be included in the emulsion system to achieve good results.

(b) Carbowaxes

Carbowaxes act as non-ionic emulsifying agents and mainly used in the preparation of ointments and creams. Their molecular weight varies from 200 to 1000. Carbowax 200 to 700 are viscous, light coloured hygroscopic liquids whereas carbowax with molecular weight 1000 and above are wax like solids. A product with desired consistency can be produced by using suitable carbowaxes.

(c) Lecithins

Lecithin forms W/O emulsions but is rarely used as emulsifying agent because it darkens in colour when exposed to light and gets easily oxidised.

HYDROPHILE-LIPOPHILE BALANCE (HLB)

Griffin (1954) devised a useful system of classification of non-ionic surfactants related to their behavior and their solubility in water. Thus providing a particular type of emulsion. The numerical values, called the Hydrophile-Lipophile Balance (HLB), denote the relative affinity for oil and water. Oil soluble materials have low values while water-soluble materials have high values. Commonly used emulsifying agents have HLB values ranging form 1 to 40. Emulsifying agents with high HLB values i.e. 7 to 20 produce O/W emulsions (hydrophilic) and those with low HLB values i.e. 3 to 6 produce W/O emulsion (lipophilic)

The following table indicates the HLB values and applications of emulsifying agents.

HLB values of emulsifying agents and their applications

Name of the emulsifying agent	HLB value	Applications	Type of emulsion
1. Acacia	8.0	Emulsifying agent	O/W
2. Glyceryl monostearate	3.8	Emulsifying agent	W/O
3. Sorbitan monooleate	4.3	Emulsifying agent	W/O
4. Sorbitan monostearate	4.7	Emulsifying agent	W/O
5. Polysorbate 20	16.7	Solubilising agent	—
6. Polysorbate 60	14.9	Detergent	—
7. Polysorbate 80	15.0	Solubilising agent	—
8. Sodium lauryl sulphate	40.0	Emulsifying agent	O/W
9. Sodium oleate	18.0	Solubilising agent	—
10. Tragacanth	13.2	Emulsifying agent	O/W
11. Triethanolamine oleate	12.0	Emulsifying agent	O/W

Choice of Emulsifying Agents

To get an emulsion of required properties, the emulsifying agent selected must have the following qualities.

1. It should be capable of reducing the interfacial tension between the two immiscible liquids.
2. It should be capable of keeping the globules of dispersed liquid distributed indefinitely throughout the dispersion medium.
3. It should be non-toxic.
4. The odour and taste should be compatible with the preparation.
5. It should be chemically compatible with other ingredients of the preparation.
6. It should be able to produce and maintain the required consistency of the preparation.

Preparation of Emulsions

For small-scale work emulsions can be prepared by the following methods:

(a) Dry gum method
(b) Wet gum method
(c) Bottle method.

In dry gum method the oil is first triturated with gum and then water is added to make a primary emulsion whereas in wet gum method the gum is first triturated with water to form a mucilage and then oil is incorporated in small quantities with constant trituration to form a primary emulsion.

For extemporaneous compounding of emulsions by dry gum method and wet gum method the most efficient apparatus used is mortar and pestle. The mortar should be flat bottomed and rough on the inner surface so as to produce fine particles of the dispersed globules. Glass mortars should not be used because of their smooth surface.

Table given below shows the proportions of oil, water and gum acacia required for fixed oils and volatile oils for the preparation of primary emulsion.

Proportion of	Oil	:	Water	:	Gum
Fixed oils	4	:	2	:	1
Volatile oils	4	:	4	:	2

The most commonly used fixed oils and volatile oils are:

- **Fixed oils:** Castor oil, cod liver oil, shark liver oil, olive oil, almond oil and liquid paraffin (mineral oil).
- **Volatile oils:** Turpentine oil, sandal wood oil, cinnamon oil and peppermint oil.

(a) Dry Gum Method

This method is also known as 4 : 2 : 1 method because these figures represent the proportions of oil, water and gum acacia required for the preparation of primary emulsion. That is, for example, if there are 40 ml of fixed oil to be emulsified then 10 gm of gum acacia and 20 ml of water or vehicle will be required for preparing the primary emulsion.

Measure the given quantity of oil with a clean and dry measure and transfer it to a dry mortar. To this add the calculated quantity of acacia and triturate rapidly so as to form a uniform mixture. Then add the required quantity of water for primary emulsion and triturate rapidly without ceasing till a clicking sound is produced and the product becomes white or nearly white. At this stage the emulsion is known as primary emulsion. Then add more of water to produce the required volume. If any soluble ingredient is also to be incorporated, that must be dissolved in the second portion of water to be added after making the primary emulsion and to produce the final volume.

(b) Wet Gum Method

The proportions of oil, water and gum are same as for dry gum method. In this method the calculated quantity of gum is triturated with water to form a mucilage. Then the given amount of oil is incorporated in small portions with rapid trituration until a clicking sound is produced and the product becomes white or nearly so. When the primary emulsion is formed, the trituration in continued for few minutes more and then more of water is incorporated in successive small portions to produce the required volume.

(c) Bottle Method

Bottle method is used for the preparation of emulsions of volatile and other non-viscous oils. The emulsions can be prepared by both the dry gum and wet gum methods. Because of low viscosity the volatile oils require greater amount of gum for emulsification therefore the proportions for oil, water and gum for primary emulsion are 4 : 4 : 2.

In this method the oil is put in a large bottle and then the powdered dry gum is added. The bottle is shaken vigorously until the oil and gum are mixed thoroughly. Then the calculated amount of water is added all at once and the mixture is shaken vigorously until primary emulsion is formed. More of water is added in small portions with constant agitation after each addition, to produce the final volume.

Other Methods

Various homogenisers and blenders are used for preparing emulsions. Q.P. homogeniser is the most widely used hand homogeniser for extemporaneous preparations. A coarse emulsion is prepared in a mortar which is then transfered to the hand homogeniser wherein the emulsion is forced to pass through a narrow aperture under pressure and thereby the particle size of the globules is reduced. The emulsion may be passed through the homogeniser several times until a satisfactory product is formed. The reduction of particle size of globules increases with the speed of pumping.

Stability of Emulsions

Stability of emulsion means that a formulated emulsion should retain its

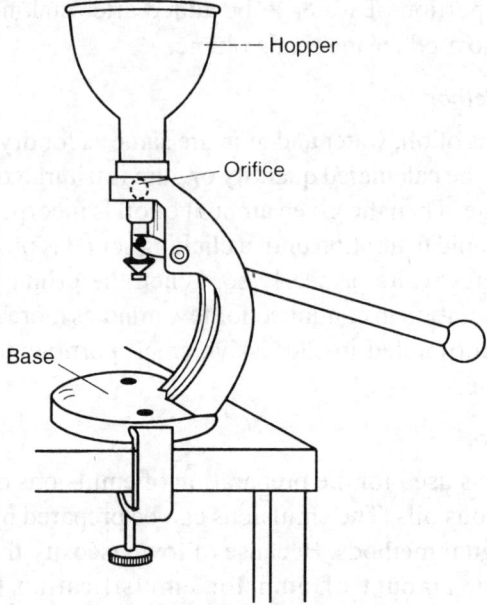

Fig. 10.6. Homogeniser.

original characters, i.e., regarding the size of globules and their uniform distribution throughout the continuous phase. Emulsions should be chemically stable and they should not allow any bacterial growth to take place.

In the present discussion only the physical stability will be discussed in detail. The three major changes associated with physical stability are as follows:

1. Upward or downward movement of dispersed globules in the continuous phase referred to as creaming or sedimentation of emulsions.
2. Aggregation of the dispersed globules forming a separate phase referred to as cracking of emulsions.
3. Phase inversion.

Creaming and Sedimentation

In creaming the dispersed globules move upward and form a thick layer at the surface of the emulsion whereas in sedimentation the dispersed globules move downward towards the bottom and form a layer over there. A good example of creaming is when milk is set aside for a few hours, a thick layer of cream forms at the surface. Creaming is a temporary phase because it can be re-distributed by mild shaking or stirring to get a homogenous product. At the same time creaming is undesirable because a badly creamed emulsion may lead to cracking with complete separation of the two phases. There are many factors which lead to creaming of emulsions but the chief factor is the rising of dispersed globules to the surface of the emulsion. The rate at which the globules will rise to the surface or the rate of creaming is governed by Stoke's law, which may be expressed as follows:

$$V = \frac{2r^2(d_1 - d_2)g}{9\eta}$$

where V = rate of creaming
     r = radius of globules
    d_1 = density of dispersed phase
    d_2 = density of continuous phase
     g = gravitational constant
    η = viscosity of the dispersion medium.

It is evident from the equation that the rate of creaming depends upon the radius of globules, the difference between the densities of the dispersed phase and continuous phase and the viscosity of the dispersion medium. Larger the size of the globules more will be creaming and smaller the size of the globules lesser will be creaming because small globules will rise less quickly than large globules. Therefore creaming can be reduced by reducing the size of globules by passing the emulsion through a homogeniser.

The rate of creaming depends upon the difference between the densities of dispersed phase and continuous phase. Greater the difference more will be creaming. Therefore this difference can be reduced but this is rarely possible in practice because it is therapeutically undesirable.

The rate of creaming is inversely proportional to the viscosity of the dispersion medium, therefore this is the most suitable approach for preparing a stable emulsion. The viscosity of the emulsion can be increased, but too high a viscosity is undesirable because it may become difficult to redisperse the materials which have settled and pouring of the too viscous product from its container may be a problem.

The high temperature reduces viscosity which encourages creaming, therefore emulsions should be stored in a cool place. Freezing should be avoided which may lead to cracking.

Cracking

In cracking the coalescence of the dispersed globules takes place and two separate layers of the dispersed phase and continuous phase are formed which are difficult to redisperse by shaking or stirring to get the original product. Hence cracking is more serious in comparison to creaming. Cracking may take place due to following reasons:

(a) By addition of emulsifying agent of opposite type

As discussed earlier soaps of monovalent metals produce O/W type emulsions whereas soaps of divalent metals produce W/O type emulsions. But the addition of monovalent soap to an emulsion prepared with divalent soap or vice versa will lead to instability and cracking of emulsion.

(b) By decomposition or precipitation of emulsifying agents

The addition of an acid to an alkali soap emulsion, e.g., turpentine liniment, leads to decomposition of the emulsifying agent with the liberation of fatty acid and alkali salt of the added acid, neither of which has emulsifying properties thus causing cracking.

The addition of sodium chloride and certain other electrolytes to sodium soap or potassium soap emulsions leads to the precipitation of emulsifying agent thus causing cracking.

(c) By addition of a common solvent

The addition of a solvent to an emulsion, which is either miscible with or can dissolve the dispersed phase, the emulsifying agent and the continuous phase leads to the formation of one phase system or clear solution thus destroying the emulsion. For example, when alcohol is added to turpentine oil liniment it forms a clear solution because turpentine oil, soft soap and water gets dissolved in alcohol.

(d) By micro-organisms

The emulsions which are stored for a long time may develop bacterial and mold growth which may destroy the emulsifying agent and cause cracking. Therefore the emulsions which are not meant for immediate use must be suitably preserved.

(e) By high temperature

When emulsions are stored for a long time an increase in temperature may reduce viscosity of the emulsion and encourage creaming.

(f) By creaming

A badly creamed emulsion is more liable to crack than a homogeneous emulsion therefore steps should be taken to retard creaming as for as possible.

Phase Inversion

In phase inversion the oil in water type emulsion changes into water in oil type and vice versa. It is a physical instability. It may be brought about by the addition of an electrolyte or by changing the phase-volume ratio or by temperature changes, etc. Phase inversion can be minimised by using the proper emulsifying agent in adequate concentration, keeping the concentration of dispersed phase between 30 to 60 per cent (higher concentration may lead to phase inversion) and by storing the emulsion in a cool place.

Instability of Emulsions

Instability of an emulsion is not due to only creaming, cracking or phase inversion but it may be due to other reasons also. Instability has been observed when the medicament is suspended in an emulsion. For example, in the case of liquid paraffin and phenolphthalein emulsion the phenolphthalein should be very finely dispersed throughout the emulsion otherwise it will settle down which will be very difficult to redisperse on shaking.

Occasionally emulsions are intentionally made with an inherent instability. An O/W barrier cream may be used which liberates a film of oil when applied to the skin. Sometimes emulsion breaking is an essential part of a manufacturing process such as the separation of wool fat from wool scouring waste.

Preservation of Emulsions

Since emulsions are prepared by using emulsifying agents such as carbohydrates, proteins, sterols and non-ionic surfactants which lead to the growth of bacteria, fungi, molds and yeasts, specially in the presence of water. The contamination of emulsions by these micro-organisms may cause unpleasant odour, taste and discolouration. The eating up of the emulsifying agent by the microorganisms will lead to changes in consistency and ultimately may cause cracking. Even if the emulsion does not crack it will become unfit for consumption. Other factors affecting growth of microorganisms in emulsions include:

(a) Deionised water and purified water if not stored properly after collection.
(b) Carelessly cleaned equipment.
(c) Type of container and closure used.
(d) The ratio of oil and water and the type of emulsion.
(e) pH of the preparation.

The above mentioned factors can be minimized to a great extent by:

(a) Using ingredients of high quality.
(b) Using boiling water to destroy the microorganisms.
(c) Using thoroughly cleaned equipment and paying particular attention to hidden parts of the equipment which are generally a major source of contamination.
(d) Using containers and closures of high quality and closures should fit well in the containers.
(e) Maintaining the prescribed ratio of oil and water.
(f) Maintaining the prescribed pH of the preparation.

The above mentioned precautions will not completely exclude the contamination therefore a suitable preservative will have to be included in the emulsion. The preservative used should have the following qualities:

1. It should be non-toxic.
2. It should be water soluble.
3. It should be effective in low concentrations.
4. It should be compatible with other ingredients of the preparation.
5. It should be effective against wide range of microorganisms.
6. It should be free from odour and taste.

Some of the commonly used preservatives in emulsions include benzoic acid, p-hydroxybenzoic acid, sodium benzoate, esters of p-hydroxybenzoic acid, chloroform, chlorocresol, and quaternary ammonium compounds, etc. Generally combinations of preservatives are used because they increase the preservation action by their synergistic effect.

Benzoic acid is commonly used for oral preparations the action of which is enhanced by the addition of chloroform as in liquid paraffin emulsions. Esters of p-hydroxybenzoic acid are popular preservatives which are used for oral as well as for external preparations. They are stable, inert, non-toxic, odourless and tasteless. They are effective against molds and yeasts, but less effective against bacteria. Sometimes the drug itself has a preservative action as in the cetrimide cream but in other preparations chlorocresol is the most suitable preservative.

Preservation from Oxidation

Substances like fats and oils obtained from vegetable and animal sources and certain emulsifying agents such as wool fat, wool alcohol and carbomer undergo oxidation by atmospheric oxygen which should be prevented by adding antioxidants. Sometimes oxidation occurs due to enzymes produced by microorganisms which should be prevented by adding suitable antimicrobial preservative.

Rx

Castor oil	8 ml
Water ad	30 ml

Fiat: Emulsio.
Signa: More dicto sumenda.
Type: O/w type emulsion for internal use.

Theory

Castor oil is a fixed oil and is not miscible with water. To make it miscible a third substance known as emulsifying agent in the ratio of 4: 2: 1, i.e., oil: water: gum will be used for the preparation of primary emulsion. Gum acacia will be used as emulsifying agent because emulsions prepared with gum acacia remain stable for sufficiently long time.

Formula for primary emulsion:

Oil	:	Water	:	Gum
4	:	2	:	1
8 ml	:	4 ml	:	2 gm

Procedure

Wet gum method

Thoroughly clean and dry a pestle and mortar. Weigh out 2 gm gum acacia and transfer it to the mortar. Measure 4 ml water and triturate it with gum so as to form a mucilage. To this add 8 ml castor oil in small quantities at a time with thorough trituration after each addition. Triturate briskly without ceasing until a clicking sound is produced and the product becomes white or nearly white. At this stage the emulsion is known as primary emulsion. Add about 10 ml more of vehicle in small quantities at a time with constant trituration so as to get a homogenous product.

Transfer the emulsion to a measure, add more of vehicle to produce the final volume 30 ml, stir thoroughly so as to form a uniform emulsion. Transfer the preparation to a bottle, cork, polish the bottle to remove finger prints, label and dispense. Attach the secondary label "Shake well before use.".

Rx

Calciferol solution	0.15	ml
Glycerin	0.3	ml
Water ad	5.0	ml

Fiat emulsio. Mitte 50 ml.
Signa: 5 ml to be taken daily.

Type: O/w type emulsion for internal use containing a small volume of oily substance.

Theory

In this prescription the quantity of calciferol solution (an oily liquid) prescribed is very small, i.e., about 3 percent. Generally speaking, emulsions containing appreciably less than 20% of oily liquid and prepared with the usual proportion of gum acacia, become unstable and readily cream. Therefore to prevent creaming, a bland of fixed oil (e.g., arachis, almond or olive) should be added to raise the total quantity of oily liquid to approximately 20%.

The substances which are prescribed in this way and require previous dilution with a fixed oil before emulsification include calciferol solution, concentrated solution of vitamin A, concentrated solution of vitamin A and D, concentrated solution of vitamin D, halibut liver oil and bromoform.

Formula for 50 ml primary emulsion:

Calciferol solution	1.5 ml
Olive oil	8.5 ml
Powdered acacia	2.5 gm
Water	5.0 ml

Procedure

Dry gum method

Take the calculated quantities of calciferol solution and olive oil in a dry mortar, add acacia powder and mix thoroughly. To this add measured amount of water, little at a time with continuous trituration until a white product is obtained and a clicking sound is produced. At this stage the emulsion is known as primary emulsion.

To the primary emulsion add glycerin with trituration. Incorporate more vehicle to dilute the emulsion. Transfer to a measure, rinse the mortar with small quantity of vehicle, add the rinsings to the measure. Incorporate more of vehicle to produce the required volume. Transfer the preparation to a bottle cork, polish, label and dispense. Attach "Shake the bottle before use." label.

Rx

Liquid paraffin	60.0 ml
Phenolphthalein	2.0 gm
Agar	1.5 gm
Acacia	15.0 gm
Syrup	15.0 ml
Cinnamon water to	180.0 ml

Make an emulsion.

Sig: One tablespoonful to be taken twice a day.

Type: O/w type emulsion containing oil and water insoluble substance, i.e., phenolphthalein.

Theory

Phenolphthalein is insoluble in liquid paraffin and water therefore it will have to be finely powdered if already not in fine powder, then mix with acacia before adding liquid paraffin and water to get primary emulsion. The final emulsion will have to be passed through a homogeniser to further reduce the particle size to get a stable and whiter emulsion because the ordinarily prepared liquid paraffin emulsions are very coarse in nature.

Formula for primary emulsion:

Liquid paraffin	60 ml
Phenolphthalein	2 gm
Acacia	15 gm
Cinnamon water	30 ml

Procedure

Finely powder phenolphthalein in a mortar. Mix it with acacia, add liquid paraffin and triturate. Incorporate cinnamon water required for primary emulsion, little at a time with constant trituration until a clicking sound is produced and a white product is formed. This will constitute the primary emulsion, the volume of which will be approximately 107 ml.

Separately in a tared dish dissolve agar in about 60 ml water by gentle heat; while hot adjust the volume to 60 ml because during heating small quantity of water will evaporate, therefore the volume is adjusted. Add syrup and cinnamon water, stir so as to get a uniform mass.

Gradually add the hot agar solution to the warm primary emulsion with constant trituration until uniform. Pass the product through a homogeniser in order to further reduce the particle size of the oil globules to get a stable and whiter product. Pass sufficient vehicle through the homogeniser to produce the required volume. Transfer to a bottle, label and dispense. Attach the secondary label, "Shake the bottle before use.".

Uses

This preparation is used as purgative.

1. Phenolphthalein is an irritant purgative which is usually given at night to act in the morning. It is administered alone or along with other purgatives such as liquid paraffin which enhances its action.
2. Acacia acts as an emulsifying agent but because of low viscosity a stable emulsion is not produced. To increase the viscosity agar is used as secondary emulsifying agent. Only a very small proportion of agar in solution can be included in an emulsion. More than 1% agar will produce a solid or semi-solid preparation, so agar must be used in proper proportion only along with primary emulsifier.
3. Syrup acts as a sweetening agent and cinnamon water as flavouring agent.

Marketed Emulsions

1. Agrol emulsion (Warner-Hindustan Division, Bombay - 400072).
   Each 30 ml contains:

Liquid paraffin	9.54 ml
Phenolphthalein	400 mg
Agar	60 mg

   Emulsifying agents and excipients to 30 ml in aqueous base containing glycerin and sorbitol solution.

2. Cremaffin liquid (Boots Pharmaceuticals Ltd., Bombay - 400038).
   Each 15 ml contains:
Milk of magnesia	11.25 ml
Liquid paraffin	3.75 ml

3. Laxol-P liquid (Medochem Labs Pvt. Ltd., Delhi - 110032).
   Each 30 ml contains:
Paraffin	9.54 ml
Phenolphthalein	400 mg
Agar-agar	60 mg

4. Magafin emulsion (Reliable Laboratories Pvt. Ltd., New Delhi - 110020).
   Each 15 ml contains:
Milk of magnesia	11.25 ml
Liquid paraffin	3.75 ml
Phenolphthalein	50.0 mg

5. Phenolax liquid (Rays Labs Pvt. Ltd., Calcutta - 700007).
   Each 5 ml contains:
Liquid paraffin	1.25 ml
Phenolphthalein	17.0 mg
Mag. hydroxide	100.0 mg

SEMISOLID DOSAGE FORMS

OINTMENTS, CREAMS, PASTES AND JELLIES

Ointments

Ointments are the soft semisolid preparations meant for external application to the skin or mucous membrane. They usually contain a medicament or medicaments dissolves, suspended or emulsified in the base. Ointments are used for their emollient and protective action to the skin. They may also be used as vehicles or bases for the topical application of medicinal substances.

The absorption of medicaments by the tissues from the ointment or other semisolid preparations applied to the skin depends upon a number of factors, e.g., properties of the drugs incorporated, properties of the bases used in the formulation, condition of the patient's skin, site of application, duration of application and degree of friction used in the application of the preparation.

Creams

Creams are thought of as ointments but usually contain a water soluble base due to which they can be easily removed from the skin. They are of a softer consistency and have a lighter body than true ointment. When applied to the skin, leave no visible evidence of their presence on the skin.

Pastes

Pastes are the semisolid preparations meant for application to the skin. They differ from ointments that they generally contain a large amount of finely powdered solids such as starch, zinc oxide, calcium carbonate, etc. Due to the presence of these substances they usually become quite thick and stiff than the ointments but are less greasy than ointments.

Since pastes are stiff they do not melt at ordinary temperature thus forming and holding a protective coating over the areas to which they are applied. They can be applied to the affected part with the help of a spatula or they may be spread on any of the dressing material and then applied. They are not removed for quite a long time. The pastes are not suitable for application to the hair because they are very difficult to remove from there.

Jellies

Jellies are thin transparent or translucent, non-greasy preparations meant for external application to the skin. They are similar to mucilages because they are prepared by using gums but they differ from mucilages in having jelly like consistency. They are used chiefly on mucous membranes for their lubricating, antiseptic or spermicidal purposes. Jellies are also used for lubricating surgical gloves, catheters and rectal thermometers. Vaginal jellies and contraceptive jellies are also commonly used.

Since jellies contain carbohydrates and lot of water as base therefore they are prone to microbial growth so they must be suitably preserved. The commonly used gelling agents for the preparation of jellies are tragacanth, sodium alginate, starch, pectin, gelatin, methyl cellulose, carbomer, polyvinyl alcohols, etc.

Characteristics of an Ideal Ointment

1. It should be chemically and physically stable.
2. It should be smooth and free from grittyness.

3. It should melt or soften at body temperature and be easily applied.
4. The base should be non-irritating and should have no therapeutic action.
5. The medicament should be finely divided and uniformly distributed throughout the base.

Classification of Ointments

Ointments may be classified as follows:

1. According to their therapeutic properties based on penetration.
2. According to their therapeutic uses.

Ointments classified according to their therapeutic properties based on penetration are as follows:

(a) Epidermic
(b) Endodermic
(c) Diadermic.

(a) Epidermic Ointments

These ointments are intended to produce their action on the surface of the skin and produce local effect. They are not absorbed. These types of ointments act as protectives, antiseptics, local anti-infectives and parasiticides.

(b) Endo-dermic Ointments

These ointments are intended to release medicaments that penetrate into the skin. They are partially absorbed and act as emollients, stimulants and local irritants.

(c) Diadermic Ointments

These ointments are intended to release the medicaments that pass through the skin and produce systemic effects.

According to therapeutic uses the ointments are classified as follows:

(i) Antieczematous Ointments

These ointments are used to remove oozing and excretion from vesicles on the skin. The drugs used are hydrocortisones, coal tar, ichthammol and salicylic acid.

(ii) Antibiotic Ointments

These ointments are used to kill the micro-organisms. The agents used are bacitracin, chlortetracycline, neomycin, quaternary ammonium compounds, etc.

(iii) Antifungal Ointments

These ointments are used to inhibit or kill the fungi. The agents used are benzoic acid, salicylic acid, nystatin, etc.

(iv) Anti-inflammatory Ointments

These ointments are used to relieve inflammatory, allergic and pruritic conditions of the skin. Generally betamethasone valerate, hydrocortisone and its acetate, triamcinolone acetonide, etc., are used for this purpose.

(v) Antipruritic Ointments

These ointments are used to relieve itching. Drugs for this purpose include benzocaine and coal tar.

(vi) Astringent Ointments

These ointments cause contraction of the skin and decrease discharges. Examples of astringents include calamine, zinc oxide, aluminium acetate and subacetate, acetic acid and tannic acid.

(vii) Counter-irritant Ointments

These ointments are applied locally to irritate the intact skin thus reducing or relieving another irritation or deep seated pain. The drugs used are capsicum oleoresin, iodine, methyl salicylate.

(viii) Ointments used for dandruff treatment

Drugs include salicylic acid and cetrimide.

(ix) Emollients

These are the preparations which are used to soften the skin. The agents include soft paraffins, cold cream and water in oil emulsion bases.

(x) Keratolytic and Keratoplastic Ointments

Keratolytic ointments are used to remove or soften the horney layer of the skin. The substances include resorcinol, salicylic acid and sulphur. Keratoplastic substances tend to increase the thickness of horney layer. The examples include coal tar.

(xi) Parasiticide Ointments

These ointments destroy or inhibit living infestations such as lice and ticks. Substances incorporated into parasiticide ointments, creams or lotions include benzyl benzoate, gamma-benzene hexachloride, sulphur, etc.

(xii) Protectant Ointments

These ointments protect the skin from moisture, air, sun rays or other substances such as soaps or chemicals. The agents which are used in protectant ointments include silicones, petrolatum, titanium dioxide, calamine, zinc oxide, etc.

OINTMENT BASES

The ointment base is that substance or part of an ointment which serves as a carrier or vehicle for the medicament. An ideal ointment base should be inert, stable, smooth, compatible with the skin, non-irritating and should release the incorporated medicament readily. Since there is no single ointment base available which possesses all these qualities, therefore it becomes necessary to use more than one ointment base in the preparation of ointments.

Classification of Ointment Bases

The ointment bases are classified as follows:
1. Oleaginous bases
2. Absorption bases
3. Emulsion bases
4. Water soluble bases.

1. Oleaginous Bases

These bases consist of water insoluble hydrophobic oils and fats. The most important are the hydrocarbons, i.e., mineral oils, petrolatums and paraffins. The animal fat includes lard. The combination of these materials can produce a product having desired melting point and viscosity. The oleaginous bases are decreasing in favour due to the reasons described below:
1. They are greasy.
2. They are difficult to remove both from skin and clothings.
3. The release of medicament is not certain.
4. If some animal fat is included it may get rancid.
5. Fatty mixture bases prevent drainage on oozing areas and also prevent evaporation of cutaneous secretions including perspiration. The water retention increases the heat in the particular areas.

Hydrocarbon Bases

(i) Petrolatum (Soft Paraffin)

It is a purified mixture of semisolid hydrocarbons obtained from petroleum. There are two varieties of soft paraffins, one is yellow soft paraffin and the other is white soft paraffin. Yellow soft paraffin is a pale yellow to yellow translucent soft mass, free or almost free from odour and taste. It has a melting point of 38°C to 56°C.

White soft paraffin is obtained by bleaching yellow soft paraffin. It is a white translucent tasteless mass and is odourless when rubbed on the skin. It has a melting point of 38°C to 56°C. White soft paraffin is used when the medicament is white or colourless.

Both yellow and white soft paraffins are used and have no noticeable action on the skin and are not absorbed. Thus they are suitable for epidermal type of preparations. Because of hydrophobic nature, aqueous liquids cannot be mixed with it but sometimes wool fat and waxes are included to incorporate aqueous liquids in it.

(ii) Hard Paraffin

It is a purified mixture of solid hydrocarbons obtained by distillation from petroleum or shale oil. It is a colourless or white translucent, odourless, tasteless mass and is used to harden or stiffen the ointment bases.

(iii) Liquid Paraffin

It is also known as liquid petrolatum or white mineral oil. It consists of a mixture of liquid hydrocarbons and may be obtained from petroleum by distillation. Liquid paraffin varies in composition according to the source of the petroleum. It is a colourless, transparent, tasteless and odourless oily liquid. It is insoluble in water and alcohol but soluble in ether and chloroform.

It is used along with hard paraffin and soft paraffin to get a desired consistency of the ointment. It is also used to levigate the substances insoluble in it.

2. Absorption Bases

The term absorption is used to denote the hydrophilic characters of the base. These are generally anhydrous bases which can absorb a large amount of water but still retain their ointment like consistency. The following are some of the absorption bases used.

(i) Wool Fat

It is also known as anhydrous lanolin. It is the purified anhydrous fat like substance obtained from the wool of sheep. It is practically insoluble in water but can absorb about 50% of its weight of water. Therefore it is used in ointments where the proportion of water or aqueous liquids to be incorporated in hydrocarbon base is too large. Due to its sticky nature it is not used alone but is used along with other bases in the preparation of a number of ointments.

(ii) Hydrous Wool Fat

It is also known as lanolin. It is the purified fat like substance obtained from wool of sheep. It is a yellowish white ointment like mass with characteristic odour. It is insoluble in water but soluble in ether and chloroform.

Hydrous wool fat is a mixture of 70% w/w wool fat and 30% w/w purified water. It is a water in oil emulsion. Aqueous liquids can be emulsified with it.

(iii) Wool Alcohol

It is obtained from wool fat by treating it with alkali and separating the fraction containing cholesterol and other alcohols. It contains not less than 30% of cholesterol. It is used as an emulsifying agent for the preparation of water in oil emulsions and is used to absorb water in ointment bases. It is also used to improve the texture, stability and emollient properties of oil in water emulsions.

(iv) Bees Wax

It is purified wax obtained from the honeycomb of bees. It is of two types: (a) yellow bees wax and (b) white bees wax obtained by bleaching and purifying the yellow bees wax. Bees wax is used as a stiffening agent in pastes, ointments and other preparations.

(v) Cholesterol

It is widely distributed in animal organisms. Wool fat is also used as a source of cholesterol. It is used to increase the incorporation of aqueous substances in oils and fats.

Advantages of Absorption Bases

1. They are compatible with majority of medicaments.

2. They are relatively heat stable.
3. These bases may be used in their anhydrous form or in emulsified form.
4. They can absorb a large quantity of water or aqueous substances.

Disadvantages

These bases possess the undesirable property of greasiness but they can be more easily removed from the skin as compared to the oily bases.

3. Emulsion Bases

Emulsion bases are semisolid emulsions having cream like consistency. These are of two types: oil in water or water in oil emulsions. Some additional amount of water can be incorporated in both the types and still retain soft cream like consistency. The oil in water type emulsion bases are more popular because they can be easily removed from the skin or clothings by washing with water. The water in oil emulsion bases are greasy and sticky, therefore they are difficult to remove from the body and clothings. Examples of emulsion bases include hydrophilic ointment, rose water ointment and vanishing creams.

4. Water Soluble Bases

Water soluble bases contain only the water soluble ingredients and not the fats or other greasy substances that is why sometimes they are known as greaseless bases. They differ from emulsion bases that the latter contain water soluble and water insoluble components. Since these bases do not contain any fats or oils, they can be easily washed with water from the skin and clothings.

Water soluble bases consist of water soluble ingredients such as polyethylene glycol polymers which are popularly known as carbowaxes. Carbowaxes are water soluble, non-volatile, inert substances. They do not hydrolyse and do not support the bacterial or mold growth. The release of medicament is rapid. Depending upon the molecular weight carbowaxes are available in different consistencies, i.e., liquids, semisolids and solids. Their molecular weight varies from 200 to 8000. As the molecular weight goes on increasing the solidity and whiteness also goes on increasing. Carbowax 200, 300, 400 are viscous liquids; carbowax 1500 is soft greasy semisolid having the consistency like that of petrolatum; carbowax 1540, 3000, 4000 to 6000 are waxy solids. A blend of different carbowaxes is used to get an ointment of desired consistency.

Certain other substances which are used as water soluble bases include tragacanth, gelatin, pectin, silica gel, sodium alginate, cellulose derivatives, magnesium-aluminium silicate and bentonite. In the true sense these substances are not water soluble but they swell up with the absorption of water.

Factors Governing Selection of an Ideal Ointment Base

A number of ointment bases have already been discussed but there is no ideal ointment base which fulfils all the requirements, since different types of bases are required for different purposes. A base suitable for normal skin may not be suitable for broken skin. Similarly a base suitable for dry skin may not be suitable for greasy skin. The factors which may help in the selection of an ideal ointment base are discussed below:

1. Dermatological factors
2. Pharmaceutical factors.

1. Dermatological Factors

(a) Absorption and Penetration

The word 'absorption' means actual entry into the blood stream, i.e., systemic absorption whereas 'penetration' means transference through the skin, i.e., cutaneous penetration.

Various experiments have been conducted by a number of scientists to study the problems of absorption and penetration which may be summarised as follows:

1. Only the ointment base penetrates deep into the tissues of the skin.
2. It is mainly medicament which is absorbed into the blood stream.
3. Paraffins do not readily penetrate the skin whereas animal and vegetable fats and oils normally penetrate the skin. Animal fats, e.g., lard and wool fat when combined with water, penetrates the skin.
4. Substances which are soluble both in oil and water are most readily absorbed.
5. Water soluble substances are more readily absorbed from water soluble bases.
6. O/W emulsion bases release the medicament more readily than greasy bases or W/O emulsion bases.

(b) Effect on Skin Function

Greasy bases interfere with normal skin functions, i.e., heat radiation and sweat. They are irritant to the skin. O/W emulsion bases and other water miscible bases produce a cooling effect rather than heating effect and mix readily with skin secretions.

(c) Miscibility with Skin Secretions and Serum

Skin secretions are more readily miscible with emulsion bases than with greasy bases. Due to this miscibility the drug is more rapidly and completely released to the skin hence lesser proportion of the medicament is required when such bases are used.

O/W emulsion bases are more readily miscible with serum from broken skin therefore they are particularly useful in weeping eczema.

(d) Compatibility with Skin Secretions

The bases used should be compatible with skin secretions and should have a pH about 5.5 because the average pH of the skin secretions is around 5.5. Generally neutral ointment bases are preferred.

(e) Freedom from Irritant Effect

Ointment bases used should be free from irritant effect on the skin. All bases used should be of high standard of purity and bases used specially for eye ointments should be non-irritating and free from foreign particles.

(f) Emollient Properties

Dryness and brittleness of the skin causes discomfort to the skin therefore the bases used should possess emollient properties that they should be able to keep the skin moist. For this purpose water and humectants such as glycerin and propylene glycol are used. Ointments containing wool fat, lard and liquid paraffin also act as emollients by preventing rapid loss of moisture from the skin.

(g) Ease of Application and Removal

The ointment bases used should be easily applicable as well as easily removable from the skin. Stiff and sticky ointments are not suitable as they may cause damage to the newly formed tissues of the skin. Therefore emulsion bases are more preferred as they are softer and spread more readily over the area to which they are applied. They can be easily removed by simply washing with water.

2. Pharmaceutical Factors

(a) Stability

Fats and oils obtained from animal and vegetable sources are liable to undergo oxidation unless they are suitably preserved. Lard, an animal fat used to be a common ingredient of ointments but it is rarely used now a days because it easily gets rancid. Soft paraffin, simple ointment and paraffin ointment are inert and stable. Liquid paraffin is also stable but on prolonged storage it gets oxidised therefore an antioxidant like tocopherol may be incorporated. Emulsions prepared with wool fat are liable to surface discolouration. O/W type emulsion bases provide a good medium for growth of microorganisms, therefore must be suitably preserved.

(b) Solvent Properties

Most of the medicaments used in the preparation of ointments are insoluble in the ointment bases therefore they are finely powdered and distributed uniformly throughout the base. Phenol, if dispersed in finely powdered state may cause blisters therefore it must be dispersed in a suitable base which should keep the phenol in solution form. Hence a base consisting of a mixture of hard paraffin, soft paraffins, bees wax and lard is used for this purpose. Similarly in the case of compound mercury ointment, olive oil is used to keep the camphor in solution form.

(c) Emulsifying Properties

Hydrocarbon bases can absorb only a small amount of aqueous substances whereas some animal fats can absorb an appreciable amount of water, e.g., wool fat can take up about 50% of water, and when mixed with other fats can take up several times its own weight of aqueous or hydroalcoholic liquids. Hence wool fat is included in the base for eye ointments.

Emulsifying ointment, cetrimide emulsifying ointment and cetomacrogol emulsifying ointment are capable of absorbing considerable amount of water, forming oil in water creams.

(d) Consistency

The ointments produced should be of suitable consistency. They should neither be too hard nor too soft. They should withstand the climatic conditions. Thus in summer they should not become too soft and in winter not too hard to be difficult to remove from the container and spread on the skin.

The consistency of an ointment can be adjusted by incorporating a suitable proportion of high melting point substances like hard paraffin, bees wax, etc., in too soft ointment; and low melting point substances like liquid paraffin in too hard ointments respectively.

Preparation of Ointments

There are two methods of preparation of ointments for extemporaneous compounding:
1. Trituration method
2. Fusion method.

1. Trituration Method

It is the most commonly and widely used method for the extemporaneous preparation of ointments. The medicaments which are to be incorporated in the base are generally insoluble in it, therefore it becomes necessary to reduce the medicament to fine powder otherwise the distribution of the medicament into the base will not be uniform.

In order to obtain the best results the medicament(s) is triturated with a small amount of the base on an ointment slab with the help of a stainless steel spatula with long broad blade. To this the additional quantities of the base are incorporated and triturated until the medicament(s) is homogeneously mixed with the base. To remove the gritty particles the ointment should be passed through an ointment mill.

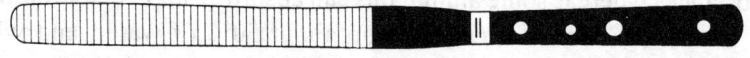

Fig. 10.7. Spatula.

When large volumes of liquids are to be incorporated, pestle and mortar should be used for the purpose. Relatively large amount of liquids can be incorporated by adding them gradually to an absorption base and then adding the fatty base. The pestle and mortar method is not as efficient as the slab method because:
(a) Certain particles have a tendency to slip out from under the pestle and thus the effect is not so pronounced.
(b) The sides of pestle and mortar will have to be scrapped from time to time.

Rx

Calamine, finely sifted	15 gm
White soft paraffin	85 gm

Label: The calamine ointment prepared by trituration method.

Procedure

Pass the calamine through a very fine sieve to get a fine powder. Triturate the calamine with a portion of white soft paraffin on an ointment slab with ointment spatula, until smooth. Gradually add the remainder of white soft paraffin with continuous trituration until a uniform ointment is obtained.

Pack the ointment in a wide mouth container or in an ointment jar, label and dispense. The container must be labelled with directions "For external use only.".

Uses

Calamine has a mild astringent action on the skin and is used in ointments to relieve discomfort of dermatitis.

2. Fusion Method

When an ointment base contains a number of solid ingredients such as white bees wax, cetyl alcohol, stearyl alcohol, stearic acid, hard paraffin, etc., as components of the base, it is necessary to melt them. The melting of the substances should be done in the decreasing order of their melting points, i.e., the substance with highest melting point should be melted first, then the substances with next melting point and so on. This will avoid the overheating of substances having low melting points. The medicament is then added slowly in the melted ingredients and stirred thoroughly until the mass cools down and a homogenous product is formed.

If any liquid or aqueous substance is also to be incorporated, that must be heated to about the same temperature as the melted bases. If it is not done so, then upon mixing the two portions the waxes or the solids will cool down quickly and they will solidify thereby they will prevent the homogeneous incorporation of the ingredients.

After melting the ingredients and mixing the two portions they should be stirred uniformly and thoroughly until homogeneous mass is obtained. Rapid cooling, i.e., by transferring into another cold container, cooling under tap water, using cold spatula or stirrer should be avoided because this will lead to the formation of solid lumps and a uniform product will not be obtained. When the ointment has begun to thicken, vigorous stirring should be avoided because this will lead to excessive entrainment of air in the ointment.

Sometimes due to the rapid cooling of the melted materials the waxy solids separate out and a uniform product is not obtained. To get a homogeneous product it can be remelted over a low heat and again stirred until cold.

Due to the greasy nature of many of the constituents of ointment bases they have the tendency to pick up dust and other foreign particles which are visible after melting the base. They can either be removed by decanting or passing through a piece of muslin which is kept in a warmed funnel or strainer and the clarified liquid is collected in another hot container.

Rx

Cetrimide	1 gm
Cetostearyl alcohol	10 gm
White soft paraffin	10 gm
Liquid paraffin	29 gm
Purified water	50 gm

Make an ointment.

Label: The antiseptic cream.

Type: Cream prepared by fusion method.

Procedure

Melt cetostearyl alcohol, white soft paraffin and liquid paraffin together. Separately dissolve cetrimide in purified water and warm it to almost same temperature (about 60°C) as that of melted substances. Add the warmed aqueous liquid to the melted mixture and stir thoroughly until cold. Pack in suitable container, label and dispense.

Uses

It is used as an antiseptic cream for the treatment of wounds and burns; for the pre-operative cleansing of the skin and for the removal of scabs and crusts in skin diseases.

Cetrimide is a quaternary ammonium compound. It is relatively non-toxic antiseptic with detergent properties. It is quite effective against gram-positive micro-organisms but less effective against gram-negative micro-organisms. Aqueous solutions containing 0.1 to 1.0% cetrimide are quite commonly used in hospitals.

3. Preparation of Ointments by Chemical Reaction

Some of the ointments like strong mercuric nitrate ointment and oleated mercury ointment were prepared by chemical reaction but now a days ointments containing free iodine or combined iodine are commonly prepared by this method.

(a) Ointments Containing Free Iodine

Iodine is slightly soluble in most fats and oils but is readily soluble in aqueous solutions of potassium iodide due to the formation of molecular compounds, e.g., $KI . I_2$, $KI . 2I_2$, $KI . 3I_2$, according to the concentration of iodine present.

These complexes are not only soluble in water but they are also soluble in alcohol and glycerin. While dissolving it must be ensured that the liquid used should be non-volatile, otherwise the distributed medicament may crystallize when the solvent evaporates and these particles in the finished ointment will lead to irritation. Due to this reason sometimes glycerin is used as solvent instead of water which will not evaporate and prevent the formation of crystals.

The aqueous solutions so formed may be incorporated in absorption type bases to get an ointment. Strong iodine ointment B. Vet. C (British Vet. Codex) is prepared in this way. This ointment is used to treat ringworm infestation in cattle. Some time back such ointments were used in human beings but they badly stained the skin with deep red colour therefore were not popular. Due to this reason non-staining iodine is used now a days.

Exercise

Prepare 100 gm of strong iodine ointment B. Vet. C.
Formula:
Iodine
Wool fat
Yellow soft paraffin
Potassium iodide
Water

Procedure

Dissolve the potassium iodide in water. To this dissolve the iodine. Separately melt wool fat and yellow soft paraffin together in a container, over water bath. Cool the melted mass to about 40°C. Add the iodine solution to the melted mass in small quantities at a time with continuous stirring until a uniform mass is obtained. Cool to room temperature and pack in glass jars. Plastic jars should not be used because iodine reacts with certain plastics.

Ointments Containing Combined Iodine

Fixed oils and many fats obtained from vegetable and animal sources can absorb iodine. This is due to the presence of unsaturated constituents in oils and fats which combine with iodine.

Paraffins which are generally used for the preparation of non-staining iodine ointment, under normal conditions, can absorb only 2% iodine because they consist almost entirely of saturated compounds while most fixed oils can combine with almost an equal weight of iodine, and some others can absorb much more than this amount. Under the conditions used for preparing these types of ointments, maximum absorption of iodine is not attained, therefore the quantity of oil used is much more than the theoretical quantity.

Although these ointments are dark, greenish-black in colour but leave no stain when rubbed into the skin as they are readily absorbed and leave no stain, therefore, they are known as non-staining iodine ointments.

Exercise

Prepare 100 gm of non-staining iodine ointment B.P.C. 1968.
   Formula:
   Iodine   50 gm
   Arachis oil   150 ml
   Yellow soft paraffin a sufficient quantity

Procedure

Finely powder the iodine in a glass mortar and add the required amount in arachis oil contained in a glass-stoppered conical flask and stir well. Heat the flask at 50°C preferably in a thermostatically controlled water bath with occasional stirring until the brown colour changes to greenish-black.

Determine the concentration of iodine as stated in the B.P.C. and calculate the amount of soft paraffin required to produce a product of the required strength.

Warm the required amount of yellow soft paraffin to 40°C in a water bath. To this add the dissolved iodine with continuous stirring.

Pour the mixed mass into a warm container and allow to cool without stirring. Otherwise air will be entrapped and the product will become opaque.

4. Preparation of Ointments by Emulsification

An emulsion system must contain an emulsifying agent if they are to remain stable for sufficiently long time. Water soluble soaps were commonly used as emulsifiers for semisolid oil in water emulsions. The viscosity of ointments or creams prevents coalescence of the emulsified phases and helps to stabilize the emulsion. The addition of cetyl alcohol and glyceryl monostearate tends to stabilize the semi-solid oil in water emulsion whereas addition of polyvalent ions such as magnesium, calcium and aluminium tend to stabilize water in oil emulsions. Nearly all semi-solid creams and emulsified ointments require a combination of emulsifiers. Due to this reason a combination of triethanolamine stearate soap and cetyl alcohol is used as an emulsifier in oil in water emulsions and a combination of bees wax and divalent calcium ions is used as an emulsifier for water in oil emulsions.

The non-ionic emulsifiers like glyceryl monostearate, glyceryl mono-oleate, propylene glycol stearate, etc., are used for oil in water as well as water in oil emulsified semi-solids because they are compatible with most of the drugs. They can be used with strongly acidic salts or with strong electrolytes.

General Method of Preparation

In the preparation of ointments having an emulsion type formula, e.g., cold cream, the general method of preparation involves the melting process as well as an emulsification process.

In this method the water immiscible components such as oils, fats and waxes are melted together over water bath at a temperature of 70°C in an open vessel. Separately, the aqueous solution of all of the heat stable, water soluble components is heated to almost the same temperature as that of melted bases. Then this solution is slowly added to the melted bases, with continuous stirring until the product cools down and a semi-solid mass in obtained.

It is very important to heat the aqueous liquid to almost the same temperature as that of the melted bases otherwise high melting point fats and waxes will immediately solidify on addition of cold aqueous solution to the melted bases or vice versa, and a lumpy product will be obtained.

Other Additives in Ointments

In addition to the medicinal agent and the base other additives such as preservatives, antioxidants, chelating agents and perfumes may be incorporated in the ointment. Preservatives such as methyl paraben or propyl paraben may be incorporated to prevent the bacterial growth in the ointments which are to be stored for a long time. Antioxidants should be added whenever there are chances of oxidative decomposition of the ingredients. Similarly chelating agents can be included to prevent the catalytic oxidative degradation by trace elements. To retard the loss of moisture from the preparation, any humectant such as glycerin, propylene glycol or sorbitol may be added. Perfumes may also be incorporated to the ointments to give it a pleasant odour. A perfume blend which should be compatible with other components of the preparation should be added.

Other Related Dermatological Preparations

Creams

Creams are viscous semisolid ointment like preparations but have lighter body than the ointments. They may be oil in water type (aqueous creams) or water in oil type (oily creams). Due to the presence of water soluble bases in oil in water type creams they can be easily removed from the skin and clothings. The aqueous creams have a tendency to bacterial and mold growth, therefore a preservative must be added. Even if a preservative has been incorporated care must be taken for complete cleanliness of the apparatus used in the manufacture of creams and containers used for packing the creams. If this precaution is not observed and a cream contaminated with microorganisms is applied to the broken skin may produce infection in the patient.

Preparation of Creams

To prevent any contamination with micro-organisms the apparatus used in the preparation of creams must be thoroughly cleaned with soap and water and rinsed with freshly boiled and cooled water and finally dried in the oven. All hygienic precautions should be taken throughout the preparation and final transfer into the containers.

Containers and Storage

Creams should be supplied in well closed containers, which should prevent evaporation and contamination. They should be stored in a cool place. The collapsible tubes made of metals or plastics are most suitable for packing the creams. Ointment jars can also be used. Aluminium tubes are not suitable for packing creams which are preserved with an organic mercury compound.

Marketed Creams

1. Betnovate-N skin cream (Glaxo India Ltd., Bombay - 400025).
   Contains:
   Betamethasone valerate   0.12%
   Neomycin sulphate   0.5%
2. Caladryl cream [Parke-Davis (India) Ltd., Bombay - 400025].
   Contains:
   Calamine   8%
   Camphor   0.1%
   Diphenhydramine HCl   1%
3. Cetrimide cream (Alpine Industries, New Delhi - 110028).
   Each contains:
   Cetrimide   5 gm
   Cetostearyl alcohol   50 gm
   Purified water   445 gm
   Liquid paraffin   500 gm
4. Dettol antiseptic cream (Reckitt & Colman of India Ltd., Calcutta - 700071).
   Contains:
   Chloroxylenol   0.8% W/W
5. Savlon antiseptic cream (ICI India Ltd., Madras - 600008).
   Contains:
   Cetrimide   0.5% W/W
   Chlorhexidine HCl   0.1% W/W
6. Silver sulphadiazine cream (Duphar-Interfran Ltd., Bombay - 400018).

Each contains:
Silver sulphadiazine   1% W/W
7. Sofradex cream (Roussel India Ltd., Bombay - 400018).
Contains:
Dexamethasone acetate   0.1% W/W
Framycetin sulphate   1.0% W/W
8. Soframycin skin cream (Roussel India Ltd., Bombay - 400018).
Contains:
Framycetin sulphate   1% W/W

Cerates

Cerates are semisolid ointment like preparations, containing a high percentage of wax which do not allow it to melt when applied to the skin. For its application they are usually spread on a material with cloth backing and then applied to the skin.

Plasters

Plasters are solid or semi-solid self-adhesive substances applied to the skin for protection, mechanical support or enhance the intimate contact between the drug and the skin. For its preparation the mass is melted and the drug is incorporated. Then the mixed mass is rolled into sticks and spread upon cloth, paper, linen or plastic. They are cut into different shapes according to the needs. The commonly used plasters are back plasters, breast plasters, chest plasters, corn plasters, and kidney plasters. Self-adhesive plaster (or tape) is the most extensively used preparation of this type. It does not require warming before application because it sticks closely to the skin at body temperature.

Marketed Adhesive Plasters

1. Adhesia adhesive plaster (Ranbaxy Labs Ltd., New Delhi - 110019).
2. Belladonna plaster (Johnson & Johnson).
3. Leucoplast (Beiersdorf India Ltd., Ponda, Goa).

Packing, Labelling and Storage of Ointments

Packing

The ointments are generally packed in ointment jars or collapsible tubes. Different shapes, types and capacities of ointment jars are used. They are made up of colourless or coloured glass. Amber coloured glass jars are used for light-sensitive preparations. While filling the ointment jars care must be taken to avoid the entrainment of air. The jars are so filled that the ointment is forced down along its sides so that no air is entrapped. Further the ointment jars are so filled to the surface that the cap or closure does not come in contact with the ointment.

Collapsible tubes made up of tin are also used for filling the ointments. For this purpose automatic machines are used. When so filled the ointments are less exposed to air, hence the chances of oxidation and contamination are reduced and preparations are likely to be more stable than the jar filled ointments. They are more hygienic because they are not contaminated by the fingers of the patient during its use. The collapsible tubes are also supplied with the applicators. So for easy application the cap can be removed from the container and applicator attached thereon.

Storage

The ointments should be stored in well closed containers and in a cool place. High temperatures are likely to soften or melt the bases during storage thereby rendering the preparation unfit for use.

Labelling

Ointment jars should be labelled with good quality of self-adhesive labels. As an additional precaution cello-tape can be wrapped around the label. Collapsible tubes should be labelled to the top because during use the tube is rolled up and this will prevent the spoilage of the label until the tube is practically empty. Self-adhesive strip labels are used because the ordinary gummed labels do not stick well to the surface of the container. Ointment tubes may be protected by placing them in cardboard boxes and the box labelled with additional label.

Stability of Ointments

The ointments should remain stable from the time of preparation to the time when whole of it is consumed.

On long storage the ointments lead to microbial growth therefore a suitable preservative must be added to inhibit the growth of contaminating micro-organisms. The preservatives must be selected very carefully. They should not react with the components of the formulations as well as the containers. Plastic containers may absorb the preservative and thereby decrease the quantity of preservative available for inhibiting or killing the micro-organisms responsible for spoilage of the preparation.

The commonly used preservatives for ointments include p-hydroxybenzoates, phenol, benzoic acid, sorbic acid, methyl paraben, propyl paraben, quaternary ammonium compounds, mercury compounds, etc. The semisolid preparations which contain water in one way or the other are more prone to microbial growth. Therefore special care must be taken regarding their preservation.

Some ingredients like wool fat and its derivatives lead to oxidation. Therefore an antioxidant may be added to protect the active ingredients from oxidation.

Incompatibilities between drugs, emulsifying agents and preservatives must be avoided. The drugs which are likely to hydrolyse must be dispensed in an anhydrous base.

Humectants such as glycerin, propylene glycol and sorbitol may be added to prevent the loss of moisture from the preparation. Pigments such as iron oxides may be added to give ointments a cosmetic like appearance particularly for those preparations which are meant for application to the face.

Ointments must be stored at an optimum temperature otherwise separation of phases may take place in the emulsified products which may be very difficult to remix to get a uniform product.

Marketed Ointments

1. Burnol ointment (Boots Pharmaceuticals Ltd., Bombay - 400038).
    Contains:
    Aminovine HCl, Thymol.
2. Ledercort 0.1% skin ointment (Cyanamid India Ltd., Lederle Division, Bombay - 400025).
    Contains:
    Triamcinolone acetonide   0.1%
3. Ledercort-N skin ointment (Cyanamid India Ltd., Lederle Division, Bombay - 400025).
    Each contains:
    Triamcinolone acetonide   0.1%
    Neomycin sulphate0.5% in vanishing cream.
4. Minit Medirub for colds (Geoffrey Manners & Co. Ltd., Bombay - 400038).
    Contains:
    Camphor   6%

Menthol	3.1%
Thymol	1.0%
Methyl salicylate	1.0%
Turpentine oil	2.0%
Eucalyptus oil	2.0%

5. Myolaxin sports ointment (Geno Pharmaceuticals Ltd., Bombay - 400008).

6. New ring-cutter ointment (Jagsonpal Pharmaceuticals Ltd., New Delhi - 110016).
   Each gm contains:

Salicylic acid	10%
Benzoic acid	7.4%

7. Scabizan ointment (Zandu Pharmaceuticals Works Ltd., Bombay - 400025).
   Contains:

Precipitated sulphur	4%
Zinc oxide	4%
Salicylic acid	9%
Benzyl benzoate	15%

PASTES

Like ointments, pastes are the semisolid preparations meant for external application to the skin. They differ from ointments that they generally contain a large amount of finely powdered solids such as starch, zinc oxide, calcium carbonate, etc. Due to the presence of these substances they usually become quite thick and stiff than the ointments but are less greasy than ointments. Due to the presence of large amount of solids they are less attractive cosmetically than ointments.

Since pastes are stiff they do not melt at ordinary temperature thus forming and holding a protective coating over the areas to which they are applied. They soothen the inflamed and raw surfaces and in particular minimize the damage done by scratching in itching conditions such as chronic eczema. It is easier to stick the pastes to the diseased areas rather than ointments which are generally less viscous than pastes and tend to spread on to the healthy skin which may result in sensitivity reactions if the preparation contains a powerful medicament such as dithranol.

Pastes are prepared in the same manner as that of ointments but when a levigating agent is to be used to mix the components and to make the preparation smooth, a portion of the base should be used as levigating agent rather than a liquid like mineral oil that would soften the paste.

Pastes were originally formulated on the principle that the high contents of powder substances would absorb exudate but it is unlikely that a powder which has been specially wetted with oil will be able to absorb an aqueous liquid.

Pastes can be applied to the affected part with the help of a spatula or they may be spread on any of the dressing material and then applied. They are not removed from the site of application for quite a long time. The pastes are not suitable for application to the scalp because they are very difficult to remove from the hair.

Zinc and salicylic acid paste which is also known as Lessar's paste is the most commonly used paste. Medicaments incorporated in zinc and salicylic acid paste are less active than when included in ointments. Higher concentrations of powerful medicaments such as dithranol may therefore be tolerated if they are combined in zinc and salicylic acid paste.

Rx

Starch, finely sifted	24 gm
Zinc oxide, finely sifted	24 gm
Salicylic acid, finely sifted	2 gm
White soft paraffin	50 gm

Make a paste. Send 25 gm.

Label: The Lassar's paste.

Type: Paste with semisolid base prepared by fusion method.

Procedure

Melt the white soft paraffin on water bath. Incorporate the starch zinc oxide and salicylic acid which has been previously sifted through sieve no. 120. Stir until cold and homogeneous paste is obtained.

Rx

Dithranol	0.1	gm
Zinc and salicylic acid paste q.s.	100	gm

Make a paste. Send 25 gm.
Label: The dithranol paste.
Type: Paste prepared by trituration method.

Procedure

Warm the ointment slab because this preparation is best prepared on warm ointment slab. Triturate the weighed amount of dithranol with a small quantity of zinc and salicylic acid paste until smooth and complete dispersion is obtained. Gradually add the remainder of the zinc and salicylic acid paste with constant trituration until whole of it is added. Check the preparation to ensure that the dithranol is completely dispersed.

Bases Used for Pastes

The bases used for the preparation of pastes are as follows:
1. Hydrocarbon bases
2. Water miscible bases
3. Water soluble bases.

1. Hydrocarbon Bases

Soft paraffins and liquid paraffin are commonly used bases for the preparation of pastes. Compound zinc paste and compound zinc and salicylic acid paste are prepared with soft paraffin base. They are used in eczema and psoriasis either alone or along with coal tar and dithranol. Coal tar paste is used for treating eczema whereas dithranol paste is used for ringworm or psoriasis. Liquid paraffin is used as a base in compound aluminium paste which is used as skin protectant.

Rx

Zinc oxide, finely sifted	25 gm
Starch, finely sifted	25 gm
White, soft paraffin	50 gm

Make a paste. Send 25 gm.
Label: Spread thickly on white lint and apply to the affected area.
Type: Paste with semi-solid base prepared by fusion and trituration method.

Procedure

Separately pass the zinc oxide and starch through sieve no. 120. Melt the white soft paraffin on water bath. Mix the required weight of powders in a warm mortar. Add small amount of melted base with continuous trituration until smooth. Gradually add remainder of the base and mix until cold and uniform paste is obtained.

Uses

It is used as an antiseptic paste.

Note:

1. Warm mortar is used because it is much easier to manipulate the paste in warm mortar.
2. This preparation is also known as compound zinc paste.

Rx

Aluminium powder   20 gm
Zinc oxide   40 gm
Liquid paraffin   40 gm
Make a paste. Send 25 gm.
Label: The compound aluminium paste.
Type: Paste with liquid base prepared by trituration method.

Procedure

Mix aluminium powder and zinc oxide in a mortar. To this incorporate liquid paraffin and triturate thoroughly until smooth.

2. Water Miscible Bases

Emulsifying ointment is used as a base for resorcinol and sulphur paste. This paste is used in the treatment of dandruff therefore it should be easily removed from the hair, hence emulsifying ointment base is used.

Rx

Resorcinol, finely sifted   1.25 gm
Precipitated sulphur   1.25 gm
Zinc oxide, finely sifted   10.00 gm
Emulsifying ointment   12.50 gm
Fiat: Pasta. Mitte 50 gm.
Type: Paste containing semi-solid base and prepared by trituration method.

Procedure

Pass separately the resorcinol, precipitated sulphur and zinc oxide through sieve no. 120 and mix the weighed quantities of these substances with a portion of emulsifying ointment until smooth. Gradually add the remainder of the emulsifying ointment with thorough trituration until smooth.

Uses

It is used in the treatment of dandruff, psoriasis (chronic skin disease in which red scaly patches develop), eczema and other skin diseases.

Emulsifying wax is used in the preparation of zinc and coal tar paste which helps in easy dispersion of the coal tar as well as easy removal from the skin after use.

Magnesium sulphate paste is prepared by using glycerin as base to which phenol is added. This paste is used for the treatment of boils because of the powerful osmotic effects of magnesium sulphate and glycerin.

Titanium dioxide paste is prepared by using glycerin and water as base. This paste is a suspension which contains titanium dioxide, zinc oxide, light kaolin, red ferric oxide, glycerin and water. It is useful for absorbing exudates from weeping skin conditions.

3. Water Soluble Bases

Water soluble bases are prepared from mixtures of high and low molecular weight polyethylene glycols. The polyethylene glycols with low molecular weight are liquid in nature whereas the polyethylene glycols with a moderately higher molecular weight are semisolid and polyethylene glycols with higher molecular weight are solids. Suitable combinations of high and low molecular weight polyethylene glycols are mixed together to get a product of desired consistency which soften or melt when applied to the skin. These bases are water soluble because of the presence of many polar groups and ether linkages.

Water soluble dental paste containing neomycin sulphate is prepared with macrogol base. Another paste contains sodium carboxy methyl cellulose, pectin and gelatin is plastibase.

Methods of Preparation of Pastes

Like ointments, pastes are prepared by trituration and fusion methods. Trituration method is used when the base is liquid or semisolid while fusion method is used when the base is semisolid and/or solid in nature. These two methods have already been discussed in detail under methods of preparation of ointments.

Preservation of Pastes

Pastes which contain water as one of the ingredients (e.g., titanium dioxide paste) or fermentable ingredients, must be suitably preserved by adding anti-microbial preservatives. They should be stored in air-tight containers so as to prevent evaporation of moisture present in the paste.

Marketed Pastes

1. Zinc and salicylic acid paste (Lessar's paste) (Agrawal Pharmaceuticals, Delhi - 110092).
2. Zinc and salicylic acid paste (Lessar's paste) (Alpine Industries, New Delhi - 110028).
3. Magnesium sulphate ointment (Agrawal Pharmaceuticals, Delhi - 110092).

JELLIES

Jellies are thin transparent or translucent non-greasy semisolid preparations meant for external application to the skin or mucous membrane. They are similar to mucilages because they may be prepared from gums similar to those used for mucilages but they differ from mucilages in having jelly like consistency. They are chiefly used on mucous membranes for their lubricating, antiseptic or spermicidal purposes. Jellies are also used for lubricating surgical gloves, catheters and rectal thermometers. Vaginal jellies and contraceptive jellies are also commonly used.

Medicated jellies contain a considerable amount of water therefore they are quite suitable as vehicles for water soluble medicaments such as local anaesthetics, spermicides and antiseptics. They are less satisfactory for insoluble medicaments which are difficult to incorporate and do not produce a uniform and smooth product.

Jellies are easy to apply and the evaporation of water content produces a cooling sensation to the skin. After evaporation the contents remaining behind stick well to the applied area and give a protection. When the treatment is over they can be easily removed by washing with water. The jellies used as lubricants for articles to be inserted into sterile regions of the body such as bladder, etc., must be sterile.

Preparation of Jellies

Pharmaceutical jellies are usually prepared by adding a thickening agent such as tragacanth or carboxymethyl cellulose to an aqueous solution in which drug has been dissolved. The mass is triturated in a mortar until a uniform product is obtained. Whenever a dark coloured drug is to be used then glass pestle and mortar must be used. For the preparation of jellies a whole gum is preferred rather than powdered gum because the former gives a clear preparation of uniform consistency. The following jelling agents are used for the preparation of jellies:

(i) Tragacanth

Tragacanth was frequently used for the preparation of lubricating, medicated and contraceptive jellies. The amount of gum required for the preparation of such jellies depends on the use of the jelly. For lubricating jelly 2 to 3% is sufficient but for dermatological vehicles about 5% gum is required. For the incorporation of ichthammol, resorcinol, salicylic acid and other medicaments a bassorin paste containing tragacanth 5% is used.

Tragacanth jellies are sometimes called bassorin pastes because the hydrophilic component of tragacanth which forms a gel in water is known as bassorin.

When tragacanth is added to water particularly, vice versa a lumpy product is obtained due to agglomeration of sticky, poorly wettable particles, which is difficult to disperse. Therefore a dispersing agent like alcohol and/or glycerin and/or a volatile oil is used to get a homogeneous preparation.

Tragacanth jellies are becoming less popular because of the following reasons:

(a) They vary in viscosity because the gum is obtained from natural sources.
(b) After evaporation the film left on the skin tends to flake.
(c) They lose viscosity quickly outside the pH range of 4.5 to 7, e.g., if benzoic acid is used as a preservative.
(d) They can't be stored for a long time.
(e) They are prone to microbial growth.

Rx

Ichthammol	1.0 gm
Tragacanth, in powder	2.5 gm
Alcohol 90%	5.0 ml
Glycerin	1.0 gm
Purified water q.s.	50.0 gm

Make a jelly.

Directions: To be spread in a thin layer over the affected part.

Procedure

To take into consideration the losses calculate for 60 gm instead of 50 gm. Take a 100 ml wide mouthed jar, put alcohol in it and add tragacanth; the reverse order may lead to lump formation. Shake well to mix. To this add water as quickly as possible and shake immediately.

Separately mix ichthammol, glycerin and 10 ml water. Add this solution to the mucilage and shake well. Adjust the final weight by adding more of water, if required, and shake well. Pack in a well closed container.

2. Sodium Alginate

Sodium alginate jellies are used as lubricants and dermatological vehicles. For lubricants 1.5 to 2% and for dermatological vehicles 5 to 10% sodium alginate is used. To increase the viscosity traces of soluble calcium salt may be added but high concentrations salt out the sodium alginate. 2 to 4% alcohol, glycerin or propylene glycol is used as dispersing agent. Sodium alginate has an advantage over tragacanth that it is available in several grades of standardised viscosity.

3. Pectin

Pectin is a very good gelling agent and is used in the preparation of many types of jellies including edible jellies. Glycerin is used as a dispersing agent and humectant in dermatological jellies. Pectin acts as a very good medium for the bacterial growth, therefore jellies prepared with pectin must be suitably preserved. Jellies must be packed in well closed containers to prevent the loss of moisture by evaporation.

4. Starch

Starch in combination with other substances like gelatin and glycerin was commonly used for the preparation of jellies. Still a product known as starch glycerin prepared by heating wheat starch with water and glycerin is used. Starch mucilages prepared with water alone lead to bacterial growth therefore a suitable preservative must be added. Glycerin in large amounts, i.e., 50% may be included which will act as preservative and humectant. Medicaments are incorporated in the cold jelly by trituration. Starch jellies should be freshly prepared and packed in well closed containers to prevent the loss of moisture by evaporation.

5. Gelatin

Gelatin is insoluble in cold water but swells and softens in it. It is soluble in hot water. A hot solution containing only 2% gelatin forms a jelly on cooling. Very stiff medicated jellies can be prepared by incorporating about 15% gelatin. Such jellies are melted before use and after cooling to desired temperature are applied with a brush to the affected area. The area is covered with bandage and the dressing may be left in place for several weeks. Zinc gelatin jelly which is also known as Unna's paste is the main preparation of this type.

Rx

Prepare 100 gm zinc gelatin jelly.

Formula:

Zinc oxide	15 gm
Gelatin	15 gm
Glycerin	35 gm
Water	35 gm

Make a jelly. Send 50 gm.

Directions: Apply to the affected part as directed.

Procedure

Soak the gelatin in water until thoroughly softened, add the glycerin and heat over water bath until the gelatin is dissolved, adjust the weight to 850 gm, if necessary, by adding more of water.

Pass the zinc oxide through sieve no. 120 and weigh the required amount and add it in small amounts to the melted base with gentle stirring to avoid excessive incorporation of air. Continue stirring until a uniform viscous product is obtained.

Pour the product so obtained in a tray to a depth of about 1 cm, with continuous trituration throughout the operation. When the mass has set, carefully cut the mass into pieces of about 1.5 cm square, with a blade or sharp knife. Pack in well closed wide mouthed container.

If the jelly is poured directly into the container, sedimentation of zinc oxide may take place if the preparation is not stirred well each time when it is used. This may result in very uneven medication if the same jar containing the jelly is used for many patients or on several occasions. Dividing the product into small pieces is a convenient method where a desired number of pieces can be melted for each treatment, which will give a uniform composition.

6. Cellulose Derivatives

Methyl cellulose and sodium carboxy methyl cellulose are widely used for the preparation of jellies. These substances produce neutral jellies of very stable viscosity and afford good resistance against bacterial growth. These jellies are quite clear due to freedom from insoluble impurities and produce a strong film after drying on the skin. Sodium carboxy methyl cellulose is used for the preparation of lubricating jellies as well as used for sterile jellies such as lignocaine gel because it can withstand autoclaving without serious deterioration.

Preservation of Jellies

Although some bases used for the preparation of jellies, e.g., clays and cellulose derivatives, resist the bacterial attack but since all the jellies contain large amount of water therefore they must be suitably preserved by adding an antimicrobial preservative, unless they are to be used immediately. Methyl p-hydroxybenzoate 0.1 to 0.2% W/V is commonly used preservative for medicated jellies.

There is quick loss of water which leads to skin formation on jellies. Therefore to prevent this a hygroscopic substance such as glycerin, propylene glycol or sorbitol may be added.

Containers

Containers containing jellies should be well filled to minimise evaporation of water, well closed and stored in a cool place to prevent drying out.

Collapsible tubes should be used for packing the sterile products such as catheter lubricants.

Marketed Gels/Jellies

1. Candid-V gel (Glenmark Pharmaceuticals Ltd., Bombay - 400026).

Each contains:

Clotrimazole   2%

2. Daktacort gel (NR Jet Enterprises Ltd., Bombay - 400078).

Each contains:

Miconazole nitrate I.P.   2% W/W

Hydrocortisone acetate   1% W/W

3. Gyno-Daktarin gel (NR Jet Enterprises, Bombay - 400078).

Each contains:

Miconazole nitrate gel

4. Gentian violet jelly (Arora Pharmaceuticals Pvt. Ltd., New Delhi - 110035).

5. Thrombophob gel (German Remedies Ltd., Bombay - 400018).

Each gm contains:

Heparin Sod.   200 I.U.

POULTICES

Poultices are also known as cataplasms. They are soft, viscous wet masses of solid substances applied to the skin for their fomentation action in order to give relief from pain or reduce inflammation or in some cases to act as counter-irritant. They are also used to draw infectious material from diseased tissues because of the absorptive and hygroscopic characters of the ingredients. They represent one of the most ancient classes of pharmaceutical preparations. Now a days the practising pharmacists never prepare poultices but sometimes may be asked to prepare such preparations. Clay metals such as heavy kaolin, herbs and seeds such as mustard, linseed, etc., are used for their preparation. Glycerin is incorporated because of its hygroscopic nature.

For use the poultice is heated in a dish with occasional stirring until the heat is tolerated on the back of the hand. Then it is spread thickly on a dressing material and applied as hot as the patient can bear it to the affected area which is sometimes first covered with muslin to facilitate removal after use. Only kaolin poultice is included in B.P. 1980.

Exercise

Prepare kaolin poultice 100 gm

Formula:

Heavy kaolin, finely sifted and dried at 100°C   52.7 gm

Boric acid, finely sifted   4.5 gm

Methyl salicylate	0.2 ml
Thymol	50 mg
Peppermint oil	0.05 ml
Glycerin	42.5 gm

Procedure

Mix heavy kaolin and boric acid with glycerin and heat at 120°C for one hour with occasional stirring, and allow to cool. Separately dissolve thymol in methyl salicylate and peppermint oil, add this solution to the cooled mixture and mix thoroughly.

Heavy kaolin is liable to be contaminated with bacterial spores like clostridium tetanii. Therefore it is necessary to heat kaolin at 120°C to kill these spores.

It cannot be heated beyond 120°C to prevent decomposition of glycerin.

Kaolin poultice is stored in well closed containers to prevent loss of volatile ingredients and absorption of moisture from the atmosphere by glycerin.

Marketed Poultice

1. Antigestine poultice (Agrawal Pharmaceuticals, Delhi - 110092).
2. Antiflamistin poultice (Arora Pharmaceuticals Pvt. Ltd., Delhi - 110035).
3. Ketolin antiplast poultice [Mehta Unani Pharmacy & Co., Rajkot - 360001, Gujarat].

SUPPOSITORIES

Suppositories are special shaped solid dosage form of medicament meant for insertion into body cavities other than mouth. They may be inserted into rectum, vagina or the urethra. These products are so formulated that after insertion, they will either melt or dissolve in the cavity fluids to release the medicament. Suppositories vary in shapes, sizes and weights. Generally suppositories weighing 1 to 2 gm are prepared. Cocoa butter or glycerogelatin is used as base.

Uses

Suppositories are used for any one of the three different purposes.
1. To produce local action.

2. To produce systemic action.
3. To produce mechanical action on the lower bowel and facilitate evacuation in the treatment of haemorrhoids, anal irritation, constipation, etc.

Suppositories are convenient mode of administration of drugs which irritate the gastro-intestinal tract, cause vomitting, are destroyed by the hepatic circulation, or are destroyed in the stomach by pH changes, enzymes, etc.

They can be easily administered to children, old persons and to unconscious patients who cannot swallow the drugs easily.

The rectal suppositories may be used for lubricating, soothing, antiseptic, local anaesthetic action or for astringent effect. Therefore they may contain antiseptics, local anaesthetics, astringents, hormones and steroids. The rectal suppositories meant for systemic effect contain analgesics, antispasmodics, sedatives and tranquilizers.

The lower portion of the rectum affords a large absorption surface area from which the soluble substances can pass quickly and reach the venous circulation directly and rapid action of the drug is produced. However the rate and extent of absorption of the drugs depends upon the nature of the base in which they have been incorporated. The maximum therapeutic effect is produced if the drug incorporated is in the finely divided state, evenly distributed throughout the base and in a readily absorbable form.

The rectal suppositories are extensively used as a mechanical aid to bowel evacuation which produce its action by irritating the mucous membrane of the rectum or by lubricating action. The glycerin suppositories are representative example of evacuant suppositories.

Types of Suppositories

1. Rectal Suppositories

These are meant for introduction into the rectum for their systemic effect. They are tapered at one or both ends and usually weigh about 2 gm. The rectal suppositories meant for children are smaller in size and weight than the adult suppositories. They usually weigh about 1 gm.

2. Vaginal Suppositories

They are also known as pessaries and are meant for introduction into the vagina. They are larger than rectal suppositories and vary in weight from 3 to 6 gm or more. The vaginal suppositories may be conical, rod-shaped or wedge-shaped. They are exclusively used for their local action on the vagina.

Special shaped suppositories are manufactured and are supplied with applicators to facilitate insertion into the vagina. Now a days a few special tablets and capsules, oval or suppository shaped are prepared for use in the vagina and are known as vaginal tablets and vaginal capsules respectively.

3. Urethral Suppositories

They are also known as urethral bougies and are meant for introduction into the urethra. They are long, thin and cylindrical forms rounded on one end. Their weight varies from 2 to 4 gm and length from 2 to 5 inch. Urethral suppositories are very rarely used.

4. Nasal Suppositories

They are also known as nasal bougies or buginaria and are meant for introduction into the nasal cavity. They are similar in shape to urethral bougies. Their weight is about 1 gm and length 9-10 cm. They are always prepared with glycero-gelatin base.

5. Ear Cones

They are also known as aurinaria and are meant for introduction into the ear. They are very rarely used. Generally theobroma oil is used as a base, prepared in an urethral bougies mould and cut according to the required size.

Newer Concept of Suppositories

Recently some newer concepts of suppositories regarding their formulation and packaging have been introduced which are described below:

1. Tablet Suppositories

Suppositories such as rectal suppositories and pessaries are formulated and prepared by compression like tablets. They contain disintegrating agents like effervescent combinations or starch. Pessaries are generally prepared as almond shape for ease in insertion and to provide a large surface area for disintegration and absorption. Rectal tablets are generally covered with thin layers of materials such as polyethylene glycol for protection and to facilitate insertion into the rectum.

2. Layered Suppositories

These types of suppositories contain different drugs in different layers. Thus the incompatible drugs can be separated from each other. Similarly drugs having different melting points or dissolution characteristics can be incorporated to control the absorption rates. These types of suppositories can be prepared by partially filling the mould with one type of material, when it congeals then the other materials are added as a separate layer and allowed to cool.

3. Coated Suppositories

Suppositories are given coatings with materials such as polyethylene glycols, cetyl alcohol, etc., to control their disintegration rate, to impart lubricant properties or to provide protective action during storage. For coating the suppositories are dipped in solutions of coating materials until coats of desired thickness have been obtained and then dried.

4. Capsule Suppositories

Soft gelatin capsules of different shapes and sizes are prepared for insertion into the rectum or the vagina. These types of capsules are increasing in popularity. Liquids, semisolids or solids can be filled in such capsules.

5. Packing in Disposable Moulds

Previously the suppositories prepared in metallic moulds or by compression method were individually wrapped and supplied in boxes. But in recent method the suppositories are directly made in disposable moulds made up of plastic materials or tin foils. The suppository mass is poured into the disposable moulds and cooled, the excess is trimmed off and the moulds are sealed, then they are packed in cartons. These types of moulds have the advantage that if due to any reason the mass melts it will remain in the mould itself which can be used after cooling.

Suppository Bases

Since suppositories are special solid dosage form of medicament they must retain its shape, solidity and firmness during storage and administration but melt or dissolve in the cavity fluids when inserted into the body cavity. Therefore the materials used as suppository bases must impart these properties and also fulfil other formulation requirements. There are a large number of bases used but theobroma oil, glycerogelatin base and poly- ethylene glycols fulfil the above mentioned requirements. An ideal suppository base should have the following properties:

1. It should be good in appearance.
2. It should melt at body temperature, dissolve or disperse in the body cavity fluids.
3. It should retain its shape when being handled.
4. It should be stable on storage, i.e., it should not undergo any physical or chemical change on storage.
5. It should be completely nontoxic and non-irritant to the mucous membrane of the body cavity.
6. It should release the incorporated medicament(s) readily.
7. It should be compatible with large number of drugs.
8. It should easily attain the shape of the mould and should not stick to the sides of the mould.
9. It should be easily mouldable by cold compression or by pouring in the cavities of the mould.
10. It should not decompose even if heated above its melting point.

Since it is not possible to get all the above mentioned qualities in a single base, so a combination of bases is used to get a product of required qualities. A number of patent "improved" suppository bases are available. Most of these are mixtures of fats, waxes and/or esters in specific proportions according to the desired qualities of the product to be obtained. Glycerogelatin and polyethylene glycols are being widely used as suppository bases, though theobroma oil is extensively used in extemporaneous preparations but it is losing its importance because it is unstable to heat and has undesirable physical properties.

Types of Suppository Bases

In general there are three types of suppository bases.

1. Oily bases
2. Water soluble and water miscible bases
3. Emulsifying bases.

Oily Bases

(i) Theobroma Oil

Theobroma oil is also known as cocoa butter. It is obtained from the crushed and roasted seeds of Theobroma Cocoa. It is a yellowish white solid which becomes white on storage. It has butter like consistency and chocolate like odour. It has a melting point of 30 to 35°C. It is a mixture of glyceryl esters of stearic, palmitic, oleic and other fatty acids.

Theobroma oil is most widely used suppository base since it melts at body temperature and release the medicament into the cavity fluids for rapid absorption. While theobroma oil is generally a very good base for rectal suppositories, it is not quite suitable for pessaries, urethral bougies or nasal bougies because after melting it has a tendency to leak out of the cavities and of its immiscibility with mucous secretions.

Cocoa butter has most of the qualities which an ideal suppository base should have but its main disadvantages are that (a) overheating changes its physical characteristics; (b) it has tendency to adhere to the sides of the mould when solidified. Polymorphism takes place when melted theobroma oil is solidified. Different crystalline forms formed depend upon the temperature of melting and rate of cooling. However a stable form is obtained if the melted mass is s allowed to cool slowly and stand for a few days in a cool place. The other disadvantages of cocoa butter are that it becomes rancid, melts in warm weather, liquefaction takes place when incorporated with certain drugs, immiscible with body fluids, failure to release the medicament and leakage from the body cavities.

(ii) Emulsified Theobroma Oil

Emulsified theobroma oil may be used as a base when large quantities of aqueous solutions are to be incorporated. Several agents have been used to form emulsified theobroma oil suppositories. The use of 5% glyceryl monostearate, 10% lanette wax, 2-3% cetyl alcohol, 4% bees wax and spermaceti up to 12% is recommended for emulsified theobroma oil suppositories.

(iii) Hydrogenated Oils

As a substitute of theobroma oil a number of hydrogenated oils, e.g., hydrogenated edible oil, coconut oil, palm kernel oil, hydrogenated pea oil, stearin and a mixture of oleic and stearic acids are recommended. Synthetic fat bases have a number of advantages over theobroma oil that:

(a) Overheating does not affect the solidifying point.

(b) They are resistant to oxidation.

(c) Their emulsifying and water absorbing capacities are good.

(d) Lubrication of the mould is not required.

(e) They produce colourless, odourless and elegant suppositories.

Synthetic fat bases also have disadvantages that (a) on rapid cooling in the refrigerator they become brittle; (b) when melted they are more fluid than theobroma oil and result in greater sedimentation of the added substances. This difficulty may be overcome by the addition of some thickening agent such as bentonite, magnesium stearate and colloidal silicon dioxide, etc.

2. Water Soluble and Water Miscible Bases

(a) Glycero-Gelatin

Glycero-gelatin base is a mixture of glycerin and water which is made stiff by the addition of gelatin. The stiffness of the mass depends upon the proportion of gelatin used which is adjusted according to the purpose for which the preparation is intended. This base has many properties that desirable suppositories can be prepared with it. The base being hydrophilic in nature, slowly dissolves in the aqueous secretions and provide a slow continuous release of medicament. This base may be used to prepare all types of suppositories but it is particularly used as vehicle in vaginal suppositories. Glycerogelatin base is well suited for suppositories containing belladonna extract, boric acid, chloral hydrate, bromides, iodides, iodoform, opium, etc.

Depending upon the compatibility of the drugs used a suitable type of gelatin is selected for the purpose. Two types of gelatins are used as suppository base (i) Type-A or pharmagel A which is acidic in nature is used for acidic drugs; and (ii) Type-B or pharmagel B which is alkaline in nature is used for alkaline drugs.

Disadvantages

Glycerogelatin base suppositories are less commonly used than the fatty base suppositories because:

1. They are more difficult to prepare and handle.
2. They are hygroscopic therefore they must be stored in well closed containers.
3. Gelatin is incompatible with many drugs, e.g., tannic acid, ferric chloride, gallic acid, etc.

4. They support bacterial and mold growth therefore a preservative such as methylparaben and propylparaben must be added.
5. The solution time depends on the content and quality of the gelatin used.

(b) Soap Glycerin Suppositories

In glycerogelatin base the gelatin is replaced with either curd soap or sodium stearate which makes the glycerin sufficiently hard for suppositories and a large quantity of glycerin up to 95% of the mass can be incorporated, further the soap helps in the evacuation action of glycerin whereas gelatin does not.

The soap glycerin suppositories have disadvantage that they are very hygroscopic therefore they must be protected from atmosphere and wrapped in waxed paper or tin foil.

(c) Polyethylene Glycols

Polyethylene glycol polymers are widely used in the extemporaneous preparations and commercial manufacture of suppositories. They are commonly known as 'Carbowaxes' and 'Polyglycols'. Depending upon the molecular weight they are available in different physical forms. Polyethylene glycol polymers having the molecular weight between 200 to 1000 are liquids and those with molecular weight higher than 1000 are wax like solids. They are chemically stable and physiologically inert substances and do not allow the bacterial or mold growth to take place. Suppositories of varying melting points and solubilities can be prepared by using a blend of polyethylene glycols of different molecular weights.

3. Emulsifying Bases

These are synthetic bases and a number of proprietary bases of very good quality are available, a few of which are described below:

(a) Massa Esterinum

This is also known as adeps solidus. It is a mixture of mono, di and triglycerides of saturated fatty acids having the formula $C_{11}H_{23}COOH$ to $C_{17}H_{35}COOH$. It is a white, brittle, almost odourless and tasteless solid. It melts at 33.5 to 35.5°C. Several grades of massa esterinum are available but grade B is recommended for general dispensing.

(b) Witepsol

They consist of triglycerides of saturated vegetable acid with varying proportions of partial esters. A small amount of beeswax is added for use in hot climates.

Suppositories prepared with witepsol bases (i) should not be ice-cooled since they may become brittle and fracture if cooled too rapidly (ii) the mould must not be lubricated.

(c) Massuppol

It consists of glyceryl esters mainly of lauric acid, to which a small amount of glyceryl monostearate has been added to improve its water absorbing capacity.

The above mentioned synthetic compounds have advantages over cocoa butter that:

1. Overheating does not alter the physical characteristics.
2. They do not stick to the mould.
3. They do not require previous lubrication of the mould rather lubrication is a disadvantage as it may spoil the appearance of the suppositories.
4. They solidify rapidly.
5. They are less liable to get rancid.
6. They can absorb fairly large amount of aqueous liquids.

Preparation of Suppositories

Suppositories are prepared by three processes: rolling, moulding (hot process or fusion method) and cold compression. The hand rolling and shaping method is of historical importance and not used now a days.

Hot Process or Fusion Method

Mould

Various types and sizes of suppository moulds are available for commercial use. In the dispensary suppository moulds with six or twelve cavities with desired shape and size may be used. For large scale production moulds up to 500 cavities may be used. They are made up of stainless steel, nickel-copper alloy, brass, aluminium or plastic.

For cleaning, lubrication and removal of suppositories the mould can be opened longitudinally by removing the screw in the centre of the plates. For cleaning, the opened plates are immersed in hot water containing detergent, then they are washed with water and dried thoroughly. Care must be taken that the inner surface of the cavities do

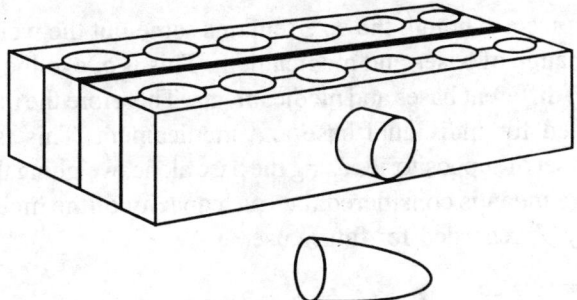

Fig. 10.8. Suppository mould.

not have any scratch otherwise suppositories with uneven surface will be produced.

Lubrication of Moulds

Whenever cocoa butter or glycero-gelatin in used as a base for the preparation of suppositories it is necessary to lubricate the mould otherwise suppositories with smooth surface will not be obtained because of the sticky nature of these bases which will stick to the sides of the mould. The lubricant applied must be of different nature than the base, otherwise it will be absorbed and fail to provide a buffer film between the suppository and the metal of the mould. Therefore an oily lubricant for cocoa butter suppositories and aqueous lubricant for glycerogelatin suppositories is useless. So a lubricant containing soft soap 10 gm, glycerol 10 gm and alcohol (90%) 50 ml is most suitable for oily bases and liquid paraffin or arachis oil for glycero-gelatin suppositories respectively.

Whenever emulsifying bases or macrogol bases are used there is no need to lubricate the moulds. Products with better surface are obtained if the mould is kept dry.

For lubricating the moulds, the lubricant should be applied with the help of a brush or a swab made of gauze. Cotton wool should not be used because it detaches the fibres too easily. Excessive lubrication of the mould should be avoided, if it happens so, the mould should be closed and inverted on a white tile to drain the excessive lubricant out.

Calibration of the Mould

Unless otherwise stated a standard mould of 15 grain or 1 gramme capacity is used, but it is not wise to assume that the capacity of the mould is correct. Though the size remains same but the weight varies with the change of bases and medicament. This is due to the change in densities of different bases and medicaments. Therefore the mould must be calibrated for individual base and medicament. This is done by preparing a set of suppositories using the base alone, weighing the product and average mean is considered the true capacity of the mould. These values may be recorded for future use.

Displacement Value

Since the volume of a suppository from a particular mould remains same but its weight varies due to the variation in densities of medicaments and the base with which the mould was calibrated. To get a product of uniform and accurate weight, allowance must be made for the change in density of the mass due to added drugs. For this purpose the displacement value of the medicament is taken into consideration.

"The quantity of the drug which displaces one part of the base is known as displacement value."

Displacement values of some medicaments used in suppositories with reference to cocoa butter are given below:

Medicament	Displacement value
Aminophylline	1.5
Boric acid	1.5
Castor oil	1.0
Chloral hydrate	1.5
Cocaine hydrochloride	1.5
Hamamelis dry extract	1.5
Hydrocortisone acetate	1.5
Ichthammol	1.0
Iodoform	4.0
Morphine hydrochloride	1.5
Phenobarbitone	1.0
Tannic acid	1.0
Zinc oxide	5.0
Liquid medicaments	1.0

The use of displacement value in calculations is described in the following example:

Prepare 10 suppositories each containing 3 grains of iodoform. The displacement value of iodoform is 4.0.

Since the 15 grain weight suppository mould is used so the total weight of theobroma oil (alone) required for 10 suppositories

$$= 15 \times 10 = 150 \text{ gr.}$$

The total quantity of iodoform required for 10 suppositories

$$= 10 \times 3 = 30 \text{ gr.}$$

4 grain of iodoform displaces 1 gr. of theobroma oil.

1 grain of iodoform displaces 1/4 gr. of theobroma oil.

∴ 30 grain of iodoform will displace 1/4 × 30 gr. of theobroma oil

$$= 7.5 \text{ gr.}$$

Therefore, the actual quantity of cocoa butter required for preparing 10 suppositories will be 150 − 7.5 = 142.5 gr.

The total weight of 10 suppositories will be 142.5 + 30 = 172.5 gr., i.e., @ 17.25 gr. for each suppository.

It indicates that although the suppositories are made in 15 grain mould their volume remains same but the weight is much more than 15 grains. Therefore it is necessary to take into consideration the displacement value of the drug while calculating the quantity of the base for suppositories.

Determination of Displacement Value of Medicaments

The displacement value of a given medicament may be determined as follows:

(a) Prepare and weigh 10 suppositories containing theobroma oil alone (or other base). Let it be a gm.

(b) Prepare and weigh 10 suppositories containing 40% of medicament. Let it be b gm.

(c) Calculate the amount of theobroma oil present in the medicated suppositories. Let it be c gm.

(d) Calculate the amount of medicament present in the medicated suppositories. Let it be d gm.

(e) Calculate the amount of theobroma oil displaced by d gm of medicament. Let it be $(a - c)$ gm.

$$\text{Displacement value of medicament} = \frac{d}{a - c}$$

Example

Determine the displacement value of a medicament in theobroma oil suppositories containing 40% medicament, prepared in 1 gm mould. The weight of 10 suppositories is 14.66 gm.

Solution

(a) Weight of 10 suppositories containing theobroma oil alone prepared in 1 gm capacity mould = $1 \times 10 = 10$ gm.

(b) Weight of 10 suppositories containing 40% of medicament = 14.66 gm.

(c) Amount of theobroma oil present = $\dfrac{60}{100} \times 14.66 = 8.796$ gm.

(d) Amount of medicament present = $\dfrac{40}{100} \times 14.66 = 5.864$ gm.

(e) Amount of theobroma oil displaced by 5.864 gm of medicament = $10.0 - 8.796 = 1.204$ gm.

$\therefore$ Displacement value of medicament = $\dfrac{5.864}{1.204} = 5$ (Approx.).

General Method of Preparation

Thoroughly clean and lubricate the mould with a suitable lubricant, keep it on ice in the inverted position to cool and drain any excess of the lubricant. The lubrication of the mould is unnecessary with synthetic bases.

Taking into account the displacement value of the medicament place the calculated quantities of powdered or shredded cocoa butter in a dish. (An excess must be calculated because of unavoidable wastage during preparation. For this the amount for two extra suppositories is sufficient, that means if eight suppositories are to be dispensed then calculate for ten suppositories instead of eight.) Heat the dish over water bath and when two-third of the base melts remove the dish from the bath and stir thoroughly until whole of the mass melts. This process prevents overheating of the base.

Place the weighed quantity of powdered medicament to be incorporated on a warmed ointment slab, over it put about half the melted base, rub it thoroughly with a flexible spatula, care must be taken to prevent the formation of lumps. Transfer the mixed mass to the dish and mix thoroughly so that a uniform mass is formed.

Warm the dish over water bath for few seconds with constant stirring until the mass becomes pourable. Transfer this melted mass rapidly into the cavities of the mould kept over ice. Fill each cavity to overflowing, this is done to prevent the formation of hollows in the tops of the finished suppositories because cocoa butter contracts on cooling and hollows are formed at the top of the suppositories. While pouring the mass into the cavities it must be continuously stirred to ensure even distribution of the medicament in all the suppositories.

When the mass has just set, remove the excess of the mass with the help of a sharp knife or razor blade or a slightly warmed spatula. Keep the mould in cool place or over ice for 10 to 15 minutes. Then open the mould and remove the suppositories. If any lubricant is there, wipe it off lightly with a clean cloth.

Cold Compression Method

This method has the advantage that it avoids heat and stirring therefore it is suitable for thermolabile and insoluble drugs. It is not suitable for suppositories in which glycerogelatin is used as base and other bases in which melting is necessary. In this method the mass is prepared by first mixing the powdered drug with an equal amount of grated cocoa butter and then incorporating the remaining amount of grated cocoa butter. Allowance is made for unavoidable wastage during preparation by calculating for sufficient extra suppositories.

The prepared mass C is placed in a cylinder A of the machine which is forced to the cavities of the mould through the narrow opening D by applying pressure to the piston B or handle of the machine thus forming

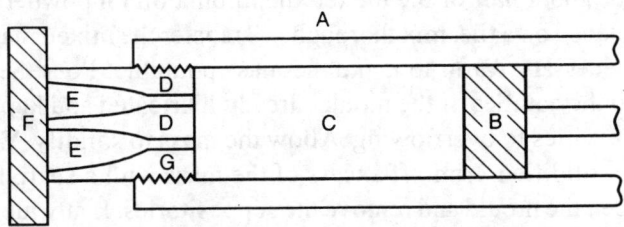

Fig. 10.9. Cold compression machine.

suppositories at E. The pressure is further applied, stop plate F is removed and the finished suppositories are taken out. The working of the machine is shown in the diagram.

The operation is repeated for the next set of suppositories. On large scale manufacturing the hydraulically operated cold-compression machines are used which are cooled by water jackets to prevent the heat of compression from making the mass too fluid.

Packing and Storage

Suppositories are usually packed in shallow, partitioned cardboard boxes which hold the suppositories in upright position and do not allow them to come in contact with each other. If plain boxes are used suppositories should be separately wrapped in waxed paper or tin foil. Glycerogelatin suppositories should be packed in well closed glass or plastic containers.

Labelling

Suppositories should be labelled with the instructions "Store in a cool place." and warning "Not to be taken orally." or "For rectal use only.".

Rx

Alum   300 mg
Theobroma oil q.s.
Fiat: Suppositorium. Mitte tales quarta.
Sig: Unus omni nocte utendum.
Displacement value of alum is 2.0.

Procedure

To take into consideration the wastage calculate for five suppositories instead of four.

Melt the calculated quantity of theobroma oil in a dish over water bath. Pour about half of the melted theobroma oil on powdered alum already placed on a tile, mix thoroughly. Transfer the mixed mass to the dish, if necessary warm to make the mass pourable. Pour the melted mass into the cavities of the mould already lubricated and kept on ice. Fill five cavities to overflowing. Allow the mass to solidify. When the mass has solidified, trim off excess of the mass with a sharp blade or knife. Open the mould and remove the suppositories. If any lubricant is present wipe it off with filter paper or clean cloth. Wrap the suppositories individually in wax paper and then pack in partitioned cardboard boxes.

Uses

Alum suppositories are used as an astringent.

Rx

Hamamelis dry extract 200 mg
Theobroma oil q.s.
Fiat: Suppositorium. Mitte tales sex.
Signa: Unum nocte si opus sit utendum.
Displacement value of hamamelis dry extract is 1.5.

Procedure

To take into consideration the wastage calculate for eight suppositories instead of six.

Melt the calculated amount of theobroma oil in a dish over water bath. Pour about half of the melted theobroma oil on hamamelis dry extract already placed on a tile, mix thoroughly. Transfer the mixed mass to the dish, if necessary warm to make the mass pourable. Pour the melted mass into the cavities of the mould already lubricated and kept on ice. Fill five cavities to overflowing. Allow the mass to solidify. When the mass has solidified, trim off excess of the mass with a sharp blade or knife. Open the mould, remove the suppositories. If any lubricant is present, wipe it off with filter paper or clean cloth. Wrap the suppositories individually in wax paper and then pack in partitioned cardboard boxes.

Uses

These suppositories are used in the treatment of haemorrhoids.

Evaluation of Suppositories

Every batch of suppositories manufactured by moulding or by compression methods must be tested to ensure that the required standards are met or not. Each suppository must be visually examined for general appearance. The suppositories containing the medicaments in suspension form should be sliced longitudinally to determine uniform distribution of the medicament throughout the suppository. Assays for active medicaments must be carried out to ensure that they conform to labelled amounts of drugs or not.

The other tests which must be performed on suppositories include:
1. Uniformity of weight test.

2. Melting range test.
3. Liquefaction or softening time test.
4. Breaking test.
5. Disintegration/dissolution test.

1. Uniformity of Weight Test

All the suppositories should be uniform in weight. The weight variation may result if some cavities are underfilled and other are overfilled. To perform this test 20 suppositories are weighed and average weight is calculated. Then each suppository is weighed individually and weight noted. No suppository should deviate from the average weight by more than 5% except that two should not deviate by more than 7.5%.

2. Melting Range Test

This test is also known as macromelting range test. During this test the time taken for the entire suppository to melt is measured when immersed in a constant temperature, i.e., 37°C water bath. The apparatus used to perform this test is a USP tablet disintegration apparatus. The suppository is completely immersed in the constant water bath and the time for the whole suppository to melt or disperse in the surrounding water is noted. This test is performed for suppositories containing fatty base only to check the physical and absorption characteristics of each batch of suppositories.

3. Liquefaction or Softening Time Test

This test is performed on rectal suppositories to determine the softening time of the suppositories. During this test a glass rod is placed on the suppository held in U-tube of the apparatus immersed in constant temperature water bath. The time taken for the rod to pass through the suppository to the constriction of the apparatus is recorded as the softening time.

4. Breaking Test

Breaking or fragility tests are carried out to determine the tensile strength of the suppositories to assess whether they will be able to withstand the hazards of packing, transporting of normal handling or not.

5. Disintegration/Dissolution Test

The disintegration and dissolution times can be determined by using the same apparatus available for these tests on compressed tablets with necessary modifications in the test media. Suppositories prepared with water soluble bases are subjected to these tests.

Use of Suppositories for Drug Absorption

Generally the suppositories are used to produce local action at the site of application but many of them are also used to produce systemic effects. Drugs such as emollients, astringents, antibiotics, hormones, steroids and local anesthetics are formulated as suppositories for treating local conditions of rectum, vagina or urethra.

Rectal suppositories are mainly used for the treatment of constipation and haemorrhoids. Suppositories are also administered through the rectum to produce systemic action. A wide variety of drugs like analgesics, antispasmodics, sedatives, tranquilisers and antibiotics are used for this purpose. The drugs which irritate the gastrointestinal tract, cause vomitting, are destroyed by the hepatic circulation, or are destroyed in the stomach by pH changes, enzymes, etc., can be conveniently administered in the form of rectal suppositories.

Factors Affecting Drug Absorption from Rectal Suppositories

The rate of release and absorption of drugs from suppositories depends on the following factors:
  1. Physiologic factors
  2. Physicochemical characteristics of the drug
  3. Physico-chemical characteristics of the base and adjuvants.

1. Physiologic Factors

A number of drugs cannot be administered orally because either they get destroyed in the stomach by the digestive juices or their therapeutic activity is modified or reduced by the liver after absorption but if the same drug is administered through the rectum, the therapeutic value is retained because the drugs are directly absorbed into the blood circulation thus bypassing the liver. About 50 to 70% drugs administered through the rectum were reported to be absorbed directly into the general circulation.

The pH of the rectal fluids plays a significant role in the drug absorption. It was proved that weaker acids and bases are more readily absorbed than the stronger, highly ionized ones. As such change in pH of the rectal fluids is likely to enhance absorption rates of acidic and basic drugs. The absorption of acidic drugs was markedly increased when the pH of the surrounding fluids was decreased. The absorption of salicylic acid was increased from 12% at pH 7 to 42% at pH 4. Similarly in the case of quinine which is a basic drug the absorption was decreased from 20% at pH 7 to 9% at pH 4. This is due to the reason that quinine becomes more ionized at lower pH values.

The condition of the anorectal membrane also plays a role in the absorption of drugs. This membranous wall is covered with a continuous layer of mucous which can act as a mechanical barrier for the free passage of drug molecules through the pore space where absorption occurs.

2. Physico-Chemical Characteristics of the Drug

For the absorption of drugs it must first of all be released from the suppository and distributed by the surrounding fluids to the sites of absorption. If a drug is fat soluble the release to the aqueous fluids will be quite slow but if the drug is water soluble then it will be released at a faster rate. After the drug has been released it is distributed by the fluids to the sites of absorption. The distribution does not depend only on the nature of the drug but also depends on the presence or absence of surfactants and physiological conditions of the colon as well as the chemical nature of the solids and liquids present in it.

3. Physicochemical Characteristics of the Base and Adjuvants

Various physical and chemical properties of different suppository bases can affect absorption of drugs to a great extent. Absorption rate is faster from oily bases having lower melting points than from those having higher melting points. Since fatty bases may become hard after moulding, resulting in higher melting point which would affect the absorption.

Adjuvants included in the formulation of suppositories can affect dissolution of the drug in the fluids as well as absorption of drugs by changing the rheological characteristics of the base at body temperature.

In emulsion type suppository bases it was shown that the release of amount of water soluble drug was increased with the increase in water content of the base.

Though suppositories are considered as a good dosage form for the absorption of drugs but there are conflicting reports with respect to blood levels of drugs when administered in the form of suppositories.

The information is difficult to correlate because of different or inadequate methods for determining blood levels, the nature of the drug and the suppository base as well as the inability of many patients to retain the suppository. Blood levels of theophylline derivatives were determined by its administration in the oral, intravenous and rectal dosage forms. Rectal retention enemas and intravenous injections showed comparable results if an allowance of 30 minutes delay is made in the rectal form.

Rectum or colon is considered as a dependable site for drug absorption but all the workers do not agree to it. A study for the absorption time on six drugs namely sodium salicylate, chloral hydrate, methylene blue, atropine, morphine and sodium iodide was carried out. It was found that the first five drugs are absorbed more quickly from the rectum and produce more therapeutic effective levels than the oral route. Whereas in the case of sodium iodide the absorption is slower by rectal route than by oral route but varies from person to person. On the whole it is generally agreed that suppositories produce therapeutically adequate blood levels.

Marketed Suppositories

1. Betadine vaginal pessaries (Win-Medicare Ltd., New Delhi - 110019).
   Contains:
   Povidone iodine   200 mg
2. Candid-V-1 tablets (Glenmark Pharmaceuticals Ltd., Bombay - 400026).
   Each contains:
   Clotrimazole   500 mg
3. Dulcolax suppositories (German Remedies Ltd., Bombay - 400018).
   Each contains:
   Bisacodyl   5 mg (infants)
                      10 mg (adults)
   Suppository base q.s.
4. Imidil vaginal tablets (Lyka Labs Ltd., Bombay - 400099).
   Each contains:
   Clotrimazole 100 mg, 200 mg, 500 mg.
5. Lotril pessary (Gufic Ltd., Bombay - 400057).
   Each contains:
   Cotrimoxazole   100 mg.

Manufacture of Nostrums

Nostrums are the preparations which are made by the person(s) who recommends them. Here the pharmacist prepares or dispenses the medicinal product according to his own judgement as to the treatment of the person to whom it is to be administered and the person concerned is present in the pharmacy at that time.

Here all the standards required and quality must be maintained as required by licensed manufacturers. The manufacturing should be done in an area which is free from all sources of contamination, clean and tidy, well lit and ventilated. The area must be protected against entry of birds, insects, rodents and microorganisms.

The equipment used should be neat and clean and must not contaminate the preparation to be prepared. Raw materials used must also be of highest quality.

The staff working over there should wear clean apron, hood, gloves and face mask so as to avoid all types of contamination during manufacturing. After preparing, the product should be packed in suitable container which must be labelled immediately on which all the suitable information regarding type of product, quantity, number of doses, name of patient, date of preparation, storage conditions, etc. must be written i.e. temperature, protection from light and atmospheric moisture, if necessary shake the bottle before use.

PILLS

Pills are the small spherical or oval solid dosage form of medicament meant for oral administration. Pills were very commonly used extemporaneously prepared dosage form which are largely replaced by tablets and capsules. Pills are usually sugar-coated or tin-coated. Nowadays no formula of pills is available in pharmacopoeias. No doubt in Ayurvedic system of medicine pills are commonly manufactured.

The pills should fulfil the following requirements:

1. Solubility

The pills must readily disintegrate in the intestinal tract. Most freshly prepared pills fulfil this requirement.

Freshly prepared pills have a drawback that the internal material shrinks within the coating which cracks and breaks off during transport. This is usually prevented by a process called 'ripening' i.e. exposing the uncoated pills in hot atmosphere until quite dry and hard. Sometimes pills dried in this way become too hard and pass the intestinal tract without disintegrating.

2. Homogenicity

All the medicaments should be thoroughly and evenly distributed throughout the pill mass.

3. Uniformity in weight

All the pills should be uniform in weight so as to ensure accurate dosage.

4. Suitability of shape

In order to facilitate swallowing, pills should be round or oval. Because of smaller diameter than tablets or capsules they can easily pass through the oesophagus. Pills should not be too large or too small for easy handling and swallowing.

5. Tastelessness and elegance

Pills should be elegant to look which can be done by sugar coating **or** polishing. Varnishing can also be done but it appreciably delays disintegration.

Formulation

The pill mass may contain following ingredients:

(a) The medicinally active ingredient(s).
(b) A diluent is added when the quantity of active medicament is very small.
(c) Excipients are required to be added to form a pill mass. It includes plasticizer, adhesive, an absorbing agent, a fluid or semisolid to render the mass plastic.

Advantages of lactose as diluent

Lactose is used as a diluent because:

1. It is colourless.
2. It is soluble.
3. It is harmless.
4. It is compatible with majority of drugs.

Lactose is preferable to sucrose which tends to absorb moisture which may thereby cake.

Preparation of pills

For preparation of pills the following steps are involved:

(a) Preparation of the pill mass.
(b) Rolling, cutting and rounding.
(c) Coating.
(d) Packing.

(a) Preparation of the pill mass

1. Pass all the ingredients through a fine sieve. Mix all of them in ascending order of their weight in a pill mortar which differs from an ordinary mortar that it is smaller and shallower with rounded edges and no spout.

2. Add any liquid ingredient and triturate thoroughly so as to mix. Initially the liquid ingredient should be added in little smaller quantity than the anticipated amount. More of liquid is added with thorough mixing. During this operation the mass generally requires loosening from the sides of the mortar. For this purpose, a non-flexible spatula is used. Then the mass is removed from the mortar and kneaded in between the fingers.

(b) Rolling, cutting and rounding

The required amount of pill mass is then rolled on a flat surface of the board of the pill machine to the exact length for the number of pills required. The mass should be perfectly cylindrical otherwise the pills will be unequal in size.

Rolling is usually started beneath the fingers and continued and completed beneath the back of the cutter dusted with powder to prevent adhesion of the pills. For this purpose powdered liquorice root or kaolin is used.

The rolled pipe is then placed flat on the pill tile and cut into the desired number of pills by to and fro movements of the cutter. After cutting, the pills are usually not round. To make them round they are quickly rotated beneath a wooden pill rounder. Small amount of kaolin or French chalk powder is dusted over the pills to make them rotate easily and smoothly. The excess powder is removed by rubbing with powder paper. This procedure is necessary when the pills are to be coated with varnish or gelatin.

(c) Coating

Coated pills are elegant, more stable and protected from atmospheric conditions as compared to uncoated pills.

For coating pills, the varnish coating, sugar coating, pearl coating, gelatin coating and silver coating is done.

Enteric coating of pills

Enteric coating is done to those pills which should not disintegrate in the stomach but should disintegrate in the intestines. Such coating is used for those substances which irritate the mucous membrane of the stomach or decomposed by stomach juices and also for substances such as anthelmintics and antibiotics or for drugs which are used in the intestines.

The substances which are used for extemporaneous coating of pills, tablets or capsules include shellac, salol, stearic acid, etc. They are insoluble in acidic medium but are soluble in alkaline medium.

(d) Packing

Pills are packed in shallow circular boxes of various kinds; the most commonly used is purple-shouldered pill boxes with flanged edges. A disc of wax paper or thin circle of cotton wool is placed on top and bottom of the pills so as to prevent them from losing their shape.

The pill box is then suitably wrapped in paper which is cut so that the margin on each side is less than the depth of the box. The folded ends are turned upwards and sealed at the sides.

PASTILLES

Pastilles are solid dosage form of medicament meant for slow dissolution in mouth. Pastilles are softer than lozenges. The base used for the preparation is either glycerin and gelatin or acacia and sugar. Since pastilles are required to be dissolved slowly in the mouth for prolonged local action, therefore, the bases should be firm enough to dissolve very slowly.

For extemporaneous preparation B.P.C. recommends the use of glycerin and gelatin in which small amount of agar may also be included.

Preparation of Pastilles

There are two types of moulds used for making pastilles.

(a) Metal moulds
(b) Starch moulds

(a) Metal mould

It consists of a number of saucer-shaped pieces of metal fixed on a plate. The cavities are lubricated with liquid paraffin and filled upto the brim with melted base.

(b) Starch mould

Starch moulds are used for large scale preparation of pastilles. These moulds consist of trays measuring about 24" × 36" × 2" which are fitted with lids to which several rows of pastille-shaped vulcanized rubber are attached. The trays are filled with starch, the surface is levelled, the lid is pressed down and then carefully raised. Depressions are thus formed corresponding to the rubber shapes. The melted mass is then filled into the depressions/cavities with a special plant and then allowed to harden. The sticking starch is removed by rapid washing and pastilles dries by keeping in the sunlight.

Containers and Storage

Pastilles are singly wrapped in wax paper, metal foil or tin foil to prevent deterioration from handling or atmospheric conditions.

Uniformity of weight

Weigh 20 pastilles and calculate the average weight. No pastille should deviate by more than 15 percent from average weight and not more than one of them by more than 10 percent from average weight.

LOZENGES

Lozenges are the solid unit dosage form of medicament which are required to be dissolved in the buccal cavity to produce continuous effect on the mucous membrane of the throat. They must be hard so that dissolution is slow. In the formulation of lozenges no disintegrating agent is included rather the quantity of binding agent is increased so as to produce slow dissolution. The formulation must contain sweetening and flavouring agent. The examples include Vicks, Strepsils, Halls, etc.

They provide local action in the throat or mouth. Their active ingredients include antiseptics e.g. benzylkonium chloride, formaldehyde, etc. Local anaesthetics like benzocaine; anti-inflammatory agents like hydrocortisone; antibiotics like penicillin; and antifungal agents like amphotericin, etc. The high contents of sugar and gum produce a sticky solution in the mouth which remains sticking to the mucous membrane of the mouth thus producing prolonged action. Flavouring agents along with additional sugar are included.

Methods of preparation

(a) Compressed lozenges
(b) Moulded lozenges

(a) Compressed lozenges

These are manufactured by compression on the tablet-making machines with the following modifications:

 (i) Very high compression.
(ii) No disintegrating agent is added.
(iii) A very high percentage of binding agent along with sugar is added.

When lozenges are prepared by compression they are known as lozenge tablets.

(b) Moulded lozenges

It is a traditional method which is still used in extemporaneous lozenges e.g. liquorice lozenges and compound lozenges of bismuth.

The apparatus used for the preparation of lozenges is called lozenge board which is available in different types one of which is shown in the diagram below.

Lozenge board

Lozenge board is made up of thick hard wood and a roller of same wooden material. Two slightly tapered bars fit into the sloping groove on each side of the board above which they project to a height of the

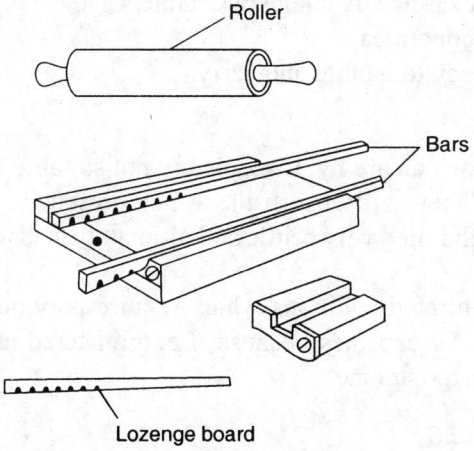

Fig. 10.10. Lozenge board.

board. Below the bars there are a number of saw cuts which fit over plates fixed across the ends of the grooves and retain the bars in the desired position.

CAPSULES

Capsules are the solid unit dosage form of medicament in which the drug(s) is enclosed in a practically tasteless, hard or soft soluble container or shell made up of a suitable form of gelatin. Hard capsules are used for filling the solid substances whereas soft capsules are used for filling the liquids and semisolids. Capsules are increasing their popularity day by day. Hard capsules come second to tablets in importance as solid unit dosage forms. Some of the capsules are administered through rectum or vagina and are convenient mode of administration of drugs than suppositories. For oral administration the capsule is placed on the tongue and swallowed with a drink of water.

Advantages

1. Capsules are tasteless, odourless and can be easily administered.
2. They are attractive in appearance.
3. The drugs having unpleasant odour and taste are enclosed in a tasteless shell.
4. They can be filled quickly and conveniently. Therefore the physician can change the dose and combination of drugs to suit the individual patient. This is an advantage over tablets.
5. They are economical.
6. They are easy to handle and carry.

Disadvantages

1. The drugs which are hygroscopic are not suitable for filling into capsules. They will absorb the water present in capsule shell rendering the shell very brittle and ultimately lead to crumble into pieces.
2. The concentrated solutions which require previous dilution are unsuitable for capsules because if administered as such lead to irritation in the stomach.

HARD CAPSULES

Hard capsules are usually made up of a base containing plasticizers and water. The base may also contain preservatives, colours, flavours and sugars. Capsule shells are made up of two cylindrical halves, one slightly large in diameter but shorter in length and the other slightly shorter in diameter and longer in length. The former is known as cap and latter as body of the capsule. The drug is filled in the narrower and longer half over which the other half is fitted as a cap.

Filling of Hard Capsules

Capsule shells are supplied in a number of sizes. The number varies from 000 to 5, the former being the largest and latter the smallest. The exact amount of a medicament which can be filled in a particular size of capsule shell depends upon density of the material to be filled in. Generally the capacity varies from 600 mg to 30 mg.

For extemporaneous filling of a small number of capsules, the proper size of the capsule shell is selected which depends upon the quantity and density of the powder to be filled in. 5 to 10% excess of each ingredient is calculated just to compensate for the loss of material which remains sticking to the pestle, the mortar and any other surfaces which come in contact during the operation. The usual procedure is that each ingredient is weighed and finely powdered if already not in a fine powder. They are mixed together by trituration so that a uniform powder is obtained. The mixed powder is placed on a paper and spread with spatula so as to make a small pile. Remove the cap from the capsule and hold it in the left hand, press the body repeatedly into the powder until it is filled. Insert the cap on the body and weigh the capsule. While weighing, each capsule of the same size must be kept in the other pan as a tare so as to get the exact quantity of drug filled in. If there are large variations

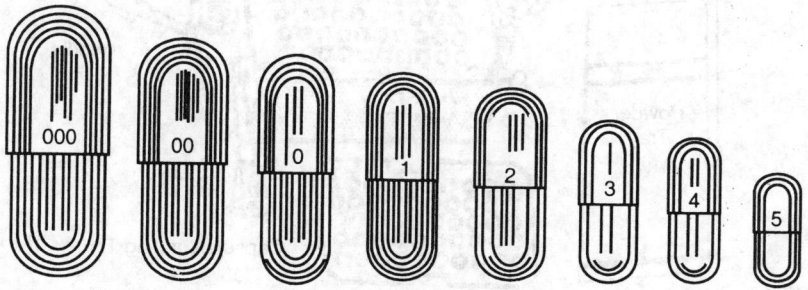

Fig. 10.11. Capsule shells.

in weights beyond permitted limits then it is necessary to repeat the process so as to fill the capsules with accurate quantity of drug.

HAND OPERATED HARD GELATIN CAPSULE FILLING MACHINE

Hand operated and electrically operated machines are in practice for filling the capsules but for small and quick dispensing hand operated machines are quite economical. A hand operated hard gelatin capsule filling machine consists of the following parts:

1. A bed with 200 or 300 holes.
2. A capsule loading tray.
3. A powder tray.
4. A pin plate having 200 or 300 pins corresponding to the number of holes in the bed and capsule loading tray.
5. A lever.
6. A handle.
7. A plate fitted with rubber top.

All parts of the machine are made up of stainless steel. The machines

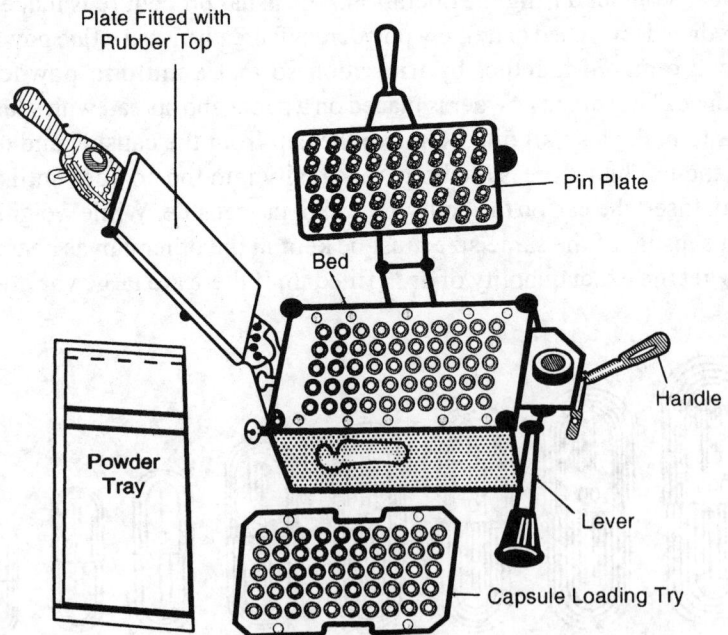

Fig. 10.12. Hand operated hard gelatin capsule filling machine.

are generally supplied with additional loading trays, beds, and pin plates with various diameters of holes so as to fill the desired size of the capsules. These machine are very simple to operate, can be easily dismantled and reassembled. Even an unskilled worker can fill the capsules without much difficulty.

Working

The empty capsules are filled into the loading tray which is then placed over the bed. By operating the handle, the bodies of the capsules are locked and caps separated in the loading tray itself which is then removed by operating the lever. The weighed amount of the drug to be filled in the capsules is placed in powder tray already kept in position over the bed. Spread the powder with the help of a powder spreader so as to fill the bodies of the capsules uniformly. Collect excess of the powder on the platform of the powder tray. Lower the pin plate and move it downward so as to press the powder in the bodies. Remove the powder tray and place the caps holding tray in position. Press the caps with the help of plate with rubber top and operate the lever to unlock the cap and body of the capsules. Remove the loading tray and collect the filled capsules in a tray. With 200 hole machine about 5000 capsules can be filled per hour and with 300 hole machine 7500 capsules can be filled per hour.

On large scale manufacturing various types of semiautomatic and automatic machines are used. They operate on the same principle as manual filling namely the caps are removed, powder filled in the bodies, caps replaced and filled capsules are ejected out. With automatic capsule filling machines powders or granulated products can be filled into hard gelatin capsules. With accessory equipment, pellets or tablets along with powders can also be filled into the capsules. Depending upon the make and model operator and the type of the materials to be filled, a machine can fill 9000 to 1,50,000 capsules per hour.

Since the primary reason of filling the drug in capsules is to avoid odour and taste of the drug, the whole aim is lost even if a small amount of the drug remains sticking outside the capsules. Therefore all the capsules whether filled by hand or by machine must be thoroughly cleaned. Small quantities of capsules can be cleaned by wiping each capsule with surgical gauze or clean cloth. On large scale they can be rolled lightly in the folds of a clean towel or cloth forward and backward until cleaned. Still another method is to rotate or shake gently the capsules with granular sodium chloride contained in a container. Then the sticking sodium chloride is removed by rolling them on a clean cloth surface.

The cleaned capsules may be polished by rolling them in a towel which has been previously sprinkled lightly with liquid paraffin. This gives very good shine to the capsules.

Difficulties in Filling the Capsules

1. Deliquescent or Hygroscopic Powders

A gelatin capsule contains water which is extracted or taken up by a hygroscopic drug and renders the capsule very brittle which leads to cracking of the capsule. The addition of an absorbent like magnesium carbonate, heavy magnesium oxide or light magnesium oxide overcomes this difficulty provided the capsules are packed in tightly closed glass capsule vials.

2. Eutectic Mixtures

Certain substances when mixed together tend to liquefy or form a pasty mass due to the formation of a mixture which has a lower melting point than room temperature. For filling these types of substances each troublesome ingredient is mixed with an absorbent separately then mixed together and filled in capsules. The absorbents used are magnesium oxide and kaolin. Heavy magnesium oxide is less effective. The use of heavy and light magnesium oxide is restricted because it forms a very hard cement-like mass which passes through the GIT without disintegration. But this type of mass is not formed when magnesium carbonate is used as an absorbent.

Another method in dealing with such type of difficulty is that the substances are mixed together so as to form a eutectic mixture, then an absorbent like magnesium carbonate or kaolin is added.

3. Addition of Inert Powders

When the quantity of the drug to be filled in capsules is very small and it is not possible to fill this much small amount in capsules then inert substance or a diluent is added so as to increase the bulk of the powder which can be filled easily in capsules. Generally smallest capsule requires at least 65 mg of the substance to fill it.

4. Filling of Granular Powders

Some powders which lack adhesiveness and most granular powders are difficult to fill in the capsules by punch method because they are not compressible and flow out of the capsule as soon as they are lifted from the pile of the powder into which they are punched. To overcome this difficulty the non-adhesive powders should be moistened with alcohol and the granular powders should be reduced to powder before filling into capsules.

5. Use of Two Capsules

Some of the manufacturers separate the incompatible ingredients of the formulation by placing one of the ingredients in smaller capsule and then placing this smaller capsule in a larger capsule containing the other ingredients of the formulation.

6. Liquids

Oils and liquids which will not dissolve gelatin may be filled into hard gelatin capsules. A measured quantity of the liquid is filled in the body of the capsule and the cap, the lower portion of which has been moistened with hot water, is placed over the body with a rotary motion so as to seal the capsule.

When the quantity of the liquid to be incorporated is small, it is first mixed with an inert absorbent which is then added to another ingredient, mixed thoroughly and filled into capsules in the usual manner.

Viscous liquids and semisolids are mixed with an absorbent like powdered glycyrrhiza so as to form a soft mass. This soft mass is cut into desired number of pieces which are then put into capsules.

Soft Capsules

These capsules are soft and elastic in nature which are prepared from gelatin and water to which glycerin, sorbitol or propylene glycol has been added as a plasticizer which make the capsules flexible. They usually contain a preservative to prevent the growth of bacteria and fungi. These capsules are available in a number of shapes and sizes e.g. spherical, ovoid, cylindrical and tubes. The spherical capsules are also known as "pearls". The contents of the soft capsules may very from 0.1 ml to 30 ml.

The soft gelatin capsules differ from hard capsules that the latter are manufactured in two steps where the shells are made on one type of machine and filling is done on another machine. Whereas soft capsules are formed and filled in one continuous operation on semiautomatic and automatic machines. They are hermetically sealed.

The capsules are used for filling liquids and semisolids. Vitamin preparations such as halibut liver oil, vitamin A and D and multivitamins are conveniently dispensed in soft capsules. They are also used for containing eye, ear, nose and throat preparations. Ophthalmic ointments are frequently packed in unit dose capsules. They are also being used as substitutes for suppositories. Nowadays soft capsules are also used for packing cosmetics, flavours and food concentrates.

Preparation of Soft Capsules

Soft capsules are generally manufactured by two methods:

1. Plate process.
2. Rotary die process.

In the plate process a warmed sheet of plasticized gelatin is placed over a plate having a number of depressions or moulds; the sheet is drawn into these depressions by applying vacuum. A measured quantity of liquid medicament is poured over it, then another sheet of gelatin is placed on it. Over this another plate of the mould is placed and the pressure is then applied to the combined plates. The capsules are then simultaneously shaped, filled, sealed and cut into individual units.

In the rotary die process, filled capsules are produced continuously and automatically. Two continuous sheets of gelatin are supplied to the two die rolls of the machine which has a number of matching dies and rotate at the same speed and in the opposite direction. As the gelatin sheets come in between the rollers the material to be filled in is injected through a metering device. The pressure exerted by the material forces the gelatin sheet to go in the cavities of the die rolls to form two halves of the capsule and fill them. The heat and pressure exerted by the die rolls seals and cuts out the capsules. The finished capsules are then passed through a series of naphtha baths to remove lubricants and then dried. These rotary die machines can produce 25000 to 30000 capsules per hour.

Packaging and Storage of Capsules

Capsules should be packed in well closed glass or plastic containers and stored in a cool place. These types of containers have advantage over cardboard boxes that they are more convenient to handle and transport and protect the capsules from moisture and dust. To prevent the capsules from rattling a tuft of cotton is placed over and under the

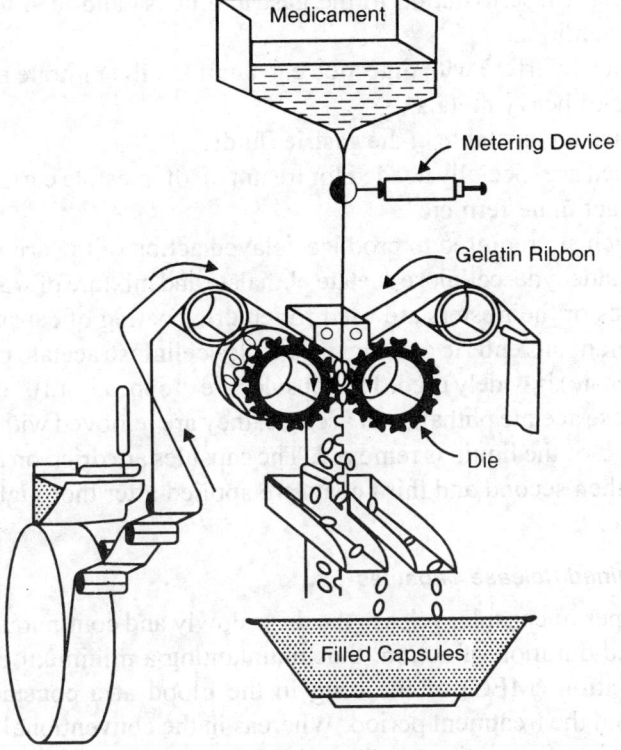

Fig. 10.13. Rotary die machine.

capsules in the vials. In vials containing very hygroscopic capsules a packet containing desiccant like silica gel or anhydrous calcium chloride may be placed to prevent the absorption of excessive moisture by the capsules. Nowadays capsules are strip packaged which provide sanitary handling of medicines, ease in counting and identification

Special Types of Capsules

(a) Enteric Coated Capsules

An enteric coated capsule does not disintegrate in the stomach or acidic medium but breaks up in the intestine or alkaline medium. They are given special type of treatment or coating which makes the medicine to pass unchanged through the stomach but set free in the intestine. Enteric coating may be given to following categories of drugs:

1. Which cause irritation to the gastric mucosa and lead to nausea and vomiting.
2. Which interfere with digestion e.g. tannins, silver nitrate and other salts of heavy metals.
3. Which are unstable in the gastric fluids.
4. Which are specially needed for treatment of intestine e.g. santonin, extract male fern etc.
5. Which are required to produce delayed action of the drug.

Formaldehyde, cellulose acetate phthalate and mixture of waxes with fatty acids or their esters are used for enteric coating of capsules. For extemporaneous enteric coating of capsules cellulose acetate phthalate (cellacephate) is widely used. The capsules are dropped in a 10% solution of cellulose acetate phthalate in acetone, they are removed with forceps and excess of the liquid is removed. The capsules are dried on a muslin strainer then second and third coats are applied after thorough drying each time.

(b) Sustained Release Capsules

These types of capsules release the drug slowly and continuously for a prolonged duration of action, thus maintaining a minimum effective concentration (MEC) of the drug in the blood at a constant level throughout the treatment period. Whereas in the conventional therapy i.e. administration of the drug in divided doses at specified intervals of time, a constant blood concentration is not maintained and there is considerable fluctuation in drug concentration.

The finely powdered drug is converted into pellets of suitable size (1-2 mm in diameter). These pellets are divided into a number of groups (generally 10 groups). The first group is kept untreated to produce rapid therapeutic effect and the other groups are coated with selected materials one by one to produce thickness of varying degrees. This can be done by giving two coatings to the 2nd group, 3 coatings to the 3rd group, four to the fourth group and so on. The total thickness of these coatings should be about 0.1 mm. All these groups i.e. coated and uncoated are then mixed together and filled into capsules. For coating, the materials may include cellulose esters, fats, keratin, gluten, mixtures of bees wax, carnauba wax with glyceryl monostearate.

(c) Rectal Capsules

Soft gelatin capsules may be used as substitutes for rectal and vaginal suppositories. Various shapes and sizes are used for this purpose. They are generally wider at one end which is inserted first, the movement of the sphincter muscles forces the capsules forward into the rectum. Liquids or solids can be filled into rectal capsules but the base in which the medicaments have been incorporated must be non-toxic, non-irritant and compatible with the capsule shell.

(d) Capsules for Packing of Ophthalmic Ointments

It is very important that the ophthalmic ointments should be sterile and free from irritant effect. Therefore, they must be packed in such a manner that the product remains sterile until whole of it is used up. The best method to keep the preparation free from contamination during use is to pack it in single dose containers. Nowadays soft gelatin capsules are very commonly used for filling ophthalmic ointments. These capsules are meant for single application to the eye. Just before application the capsule is punctured with a sterile needle, the contents instilled into the eye and the shell discarded.

Standardization of Capsules

Whether capsules are produced on a small or large scale all of them are required to pass not only the disintegration test, weight variation test and percentage of medicament test but a visual inspection must be made as they roll off the capsule machine onto a conveyor belt regarding uniformity in shape, size, colour and filling. As the capsules move in front of the inspectors the visibly defective or suspected of being less than perfect are picked out. If the number of defective capsules is large it may be due to some fault in the capsule filling machine which must be corrected.

The hard and soft gelatin capsules should be subjected to following tests for their standardization:

1. Shape and size.
2. Colour.
3. Thickness of capsule shell.
4. Leaking test for semisolid and liquid ingredients from soft capsules.
5. Disintegration test.
6. Weight variation test.
7. Percentage of medicament test.

In official books the following quality control tests are recommended for capsules:

(a) Disintegration Test

For performing disintegration test on capsules the tablet disintegration test apparatus is used but the guiding disc may not be used except that the capsules float on top of the water. One capsule is placed in each tube which are then suspended in the beakers to move up and down for 30 minutes, unless otherwise stated in the monograph. The capsules pass the test if no residue of drug or other than fragments of shell remains on No. 10 mesh screen of the tubes.

(b) Weight Variation Test

20 capsules are taken at random and weighed. Their average weight is calculated then each capsule is weighed individually and their weight noted. The capsules pass the test if the weight of individual capsule falls within 90-110% of the average weight. If this requirement is not met, then the weight of the contents for each individual capsule is determined and compared with the average weight of contents. The contents from the shells can be removed just by emptying or with the help of small brush. From soft gelatin capsules the contents are removed by squeezing the shells which has been carefully cut. The remainder contents are removed by washing with a suitable solvent. After drying the shells they are weighed and the content weights of the individual capsules are calculated. The requirements are met if (a) not more than 2 of the differences are greater than 10% of the average net content, and (b) in no case the difference is greater than 25%.

(c) Contents Uniformity Test

This test is applicable to all capsules which are meant for oral administration. For this test a sample of the contents is assayed as described in individual monographs and the values calculated which must comply with the prescribed standards.

11

Additives Used in Various Dosage Forms

Additives are the substances other than the active medicament(s) in the formulation which do not have any pharmacological action. They are used to give a particular shape to the formulation, to increase the stability and/or to increase the palatability and elegance of the preparation. Additives may be exemplified by surfactants, hydrocolloids, diluents, vehicles, bases, stabilizers, preservatives, colouring agents, flavouring agents and sweetening agents, etc. Some of the formulations may contain all the additives but others may contain one or more than one additive. They should be used very carefully so that they may not interfere with the therapeutic activity of the active medicament and does not affect the stability of the preparation.

Surfactants

Surfactants or surface active agents are one of the most important classes of additives which are used in pharmaceutical formulations. Due to one reason or the other they are used in almost all liquid, semisolid or solid formulations. They may be used as emulsifying agents, detergents, solubilising agents, wetting agents, foaming agents, antifoaming agents, flocculating agents and deflocculating agents.

Surfactants may be defined as the substances which when added to a liquid, lower the interfacial tension between two phases, thus make them miscible with each other. This phenomenon is commonly used to make two immiscible liquids miscible with each other and to dissolve the drugs which are normally insoluble in aqueous vehicles.

The molecules of a surfactant consist of two parts, i.e., a polar part and non-polar part. When such molecules are placed in two phases of different polarities the polar part moves towards high polarity phase while non-polar part moves towards the low polarity phase and preferentially they are adsorbed at the interphase. As the concentration is increased, a level is reached where the interphase becomes saturated with surface active agents and no more space is available at the surface to be occupied, therefore the surfactant molecules move towards the bulk of the solution. At this concentration an unusual phenomenon occurs. The molecules tend to form colloidal aggregates known as micelles consisting of 50 to 150 molecules of surface active agents. The concentration of surfactant at which the micelles are formed is known as critical micelle concentration or C.M.C. The solubilization begins at C.M.C. and generally increases with increase in the concentration of micelles.

Classification of Surfactants

Surfactants may be classified in a number of ways depending on the use and physical or chemical properties but the most widely accepted system of classification is based on their ionic behaviour in solutions which is explained as follows:

(a) Anionics/anion active surfactants: They ionise in aqueous solutions into a large anion which is responsible for their emulsifying ability. Examples are soaps of monovalent and divalent metals, sulphated compounds like sodium lauryl sulphate, sodium cetyl sulphate, sulfonated compounds like dioctyl sodium sulfosuccinate, etc.

(b) Cationics/cation active surfactants: They ionise in aqueous solutions into a large cation, responsible for their emulsifying ability. Examples are benzylkonium chloride, cetyl trimethyl ammonium bromide, etc.

(c) Non-ionic surfactants: They do not ionise in aqueous solutions. Examples are glyceryl monostearate, spans and tweens. This is the most widely used class of surfactants in pharmaceutical industries because they offer a wide range of physical properties and are stable over a wide range of pH.

Hydrocolloids

Hydrocolloids are the high molecular weight solid substances which when added to water produce highly viscous solutions, suspensions or gels. They are also known as gums and consist of polysaccharides, and proteins. Most of the water soluble hydrocolloids are more soluble in hot water than in cold water and tend to precipitate or form gel on cooling, e.g., agar and gelatin. Certain water-soluble polymers like methyl cellulose, hydroxy propyl cellulose are more soluble in cold water than in hot water. Their solutions tend to gel on heating.

Classification

Hydrocolloids may be classified as follows:
(a) Natural
(b) Semi-synthetic
(c) Synthetic.

(a) Natural

Naturally occuring hydrocolloids may be obtained from plants, animals and minerals. Hydrocolloids obtained from plants are most widely used and are known as gums which consist of polysaccharides. They are very commonly used in textile, paper, food, cosmetic, pharmaceutical and other industries. The hydrocolloids obtained from plants include acacia, tragacanth, agar, etc. Gelatin and casein are the examples of hydrocolloids obtained from animals. The mineral hydrocolloids include colloidal silica, colloidal alumina, bentonite and veegum.

(b) Semi-Synthetic Hydrocolloids

They are the substances which are produced by chemical modification of cellulose obtained from wood, pulp or cotton to produce soluble polymers. The modified derivatives so produced have many advantages over the parent molecules. Some of the hydrocolloids produced in this way are methylcellulose, sodium carboxymethyl cellulose, hydroxyethyl cellulose and hydroxypropyl cellulose.

(c) Synthetic Hydrocolloids

A number of hydrocolloids have been synthesised but only a few are used in pharmaceutical formulations, e.g., carbopols and polyox.

Vehicles

A vehicle may be described as a medium in which the ingredients of a formulation are dissolved, suspended or dispersed for their easy administration and rapid pharmacological action. The vehicle is a loose word which may be used for liquids, semisolids or solids. When a liquid is used to dissolve or suspend the medicament, the liquid is known as vehicle whereas when semisolid or solid is used to disperse the medicament, it is known as base. Vehicles may also by used to increase the bulk of the preparation. The commonly used vehicles in pharmaceutical formulations are described below:

1. Water

Water is the most suitable choice of vehicle because it can dissolve a large number of drugs and they can be easily administered to the body as it does not interfere with the metabolic reactions.

When water is required as vehicle for oral preparations, potable water or purified water should be used. Sometimes, potable water contains dissolved impurities and micro-organisms therefore it should be made free from impurities and must be freshly boiled and cooled to destroy the micro-organisms.

2. Aromatic Waters

Sometimes aromatic waters are used as vehicles mainly due to their flavouring properties. Some of them possess mild therapeutic and/or preservative properties. The commonly used aromatic waters are chloroform water, camphor water, cinnamon water, peppermint water, anise water and dill water.

3. Infusions

Some of the infusions which have definite therapeutic properties are prescribed as vehicles. They include compound gentian infusion, orange peel infusion, senega infusion and infusion of clove.

4. Water for Injection

Whenever water is to be used as vehicle in injectable preparations, distilled water free from pyrogens must be used. Water is used as the vehicle for most of injectable preparations because aqueous preparations are tolerated well by the body and are the safest and easiest to administer.

5. Alcohol

Alcohol is considered a very good solvent which comes next in importance to water. It has an advantage over water that preparations made with it remain stable for quite a long time because of its antimicrobial properties, while many aqueous solutions of organic substances soon hydrolyse and become unfit for use. Water and alcohol are quite miscible with each other and can be mixed in any proportions. Such mixtures of water and alcohol are referred to as hydroalcoholic solvents which are extensively used in pharmaceutical formulations.

6. Glycerin

Glycerin is an excellent solvent but it is not as commonly used as that of water or alcohol. It is a polyhydric alcohol which is quite viscous and hygroscopic in nature. Because of its viscous nature glycerin is an essential ingredient of throat paints so that the medicament should remain in contact with mucous membrane of the throat for a longer time. Due to humectant properties, glycerin is used in creams, jellies, paints, lotions and other preparations meant for external application to the skin.

7. Propylene Glycol

Propylene glycol is widely used as a substitute for glycerin. It is miscible with water, acetone and chloroform in all proportions. It can dissolve many volatile oils but fixed oils are insoluble in it.

8. Oils

Oils obtained from vegetable and animal kingdom are frequently used as solvents for pharmaceutical preparations. Vegetable oils like castor oil, cottonseed oil and corn oil are commonly used but they are decreasing in favour because they easily get rancid and develop bacterial growth on storage. They differ greatly in their qualities because they are obtained from natural origin. Due to these reasons vegetable oils are being replaced with mineral oils like liquid paraffin because it is quite stable and free from odour and taste. But liquid paraffin or solid paraffin cannot be used in parenteral preparations because they would not be metabolised by the body tissues and may develop tissue reactions and even tumours. Therefore oils are generally used in preparations meant for external use.

Some newer non-aqueous vehicles are recently developed which are used in the formulation of parenteral preparations and they are found more satisfactory than vegetable and mineral oils. Among these are polyethylene glycols, isopropyl myristate, etc.

Bases

The term base is used for semisolid and solid substances in which the drug is incorporated either to increase the bulk or to give a particular shape to the dosage form. Generally these types of bases are used for the preparation of ointments and suppositories where they are known as ointment bases and suppository bases respectively. These types of bases do not merely carry the medicaments but exert great influence over their pharmacological actions. The rate of absorption of a drug through the skin mainly depends on the nature of ointment base used in the formulation of ointments. An ideal ointment base should be non-irritant, easily applicable, easily removable, compatible with medicaments and skin secretions and should release the incorporated medicament readily. The commonly used ointment bases are soft paraffin, hard paraffin, liquid paraffin, wool fat, wool alcohol, bees wax, etc.

Since the suppositories are special shaped solid dosage form of medicament they must retain its shape, solidity and firmness during storage and administration but must melt or dissolve in the cavity fluids when inserted into the body cavity. Therefore the materials used as suppository bases must impart these properties and also fulfil other formulation requirements. There are a large number of bases used but theobroma oil, glycerogelatin and polyethylene glycols fulfils the above mentioned requirements. Coconut oil, stearin, hydrogenated peanut oil and mixture of oleic acid and stearic acid in combination with some waxes have also been recommended as suppository bases.

Diluents

Diluents are the inert substances which are specially added to increase the bulk of a drug or to decrease its concentration. The liquids which are used as vehicles may be specifically used as diluents but for oral preparations water is the most suitable diluent.

Solid diluents are included in the formulation of powders, granules, capsules and tablets, etc., where they are used to increase the bulk of other materials for easy conversion into proper dosage form. In potent drugs, diluents are incorporated to increase the bulk so that they can be weighed easily and divided conveniently into required number of doses.

The diluent used must be inert, compatible with other ingredients of the formulation, physically and chemically stable and should not affect the bioavailability of the drug. There are a large number of substances available which can be used as diluents but lactose is the most suitable and widely used diluent for oral preparations. Other diluents which are used include sucrose, sorbitol, mannitol, wheat starch, corn starch, rice starch, potato starch, and microcrystalline cellulose. Some salts like dibasic calcium phosphate, calcium sulphate and sodium chloride, etc., can also be used as diluents.

The diluents incorporated in the formulations meant of external use include talc, kaolin, starch, etc. Talc is the most widely used diluent in dusting powders because apart from diluent action, it imparts necessary spreading characteristics to the dusting powders. Whenever talc is used as diluent, sterilized talc free from cl. tetani must be used.

Stabilizers

Stability of pharmaceutical product may be defined as the capability of a particular formulation in a specific container to remain within the physical, chemical, microbiogical, therapeutic and toxicological specifications. The substances which are used to control these stabilities are known as stabilizers. The most important stabilizers are the antioxidants and preservatives.

(a) Antioxidants

An antioxidant is a substance which is added to pharmaceutical formulation to prevent the oxidative degradation of the drug. The antioxidants have great affinity for oxygen and when they are added to formulation they compete for it affording protection to other oxygen sensitive drugs.

An ideal antioxidant should be stable and effective against a wide range of pH, colourless, nontoxic, nonirritant, thermostable and compatible with formulation ingredients and packaging material. Some of the commonly used antioxidants are sodium bisulfite, sodium metabisulfite, sodium thiosulphate, ascorbic acid, ascorbyl palmitate hydroquinone, propyl gallate, butylated hydroxy toluene, butylated hydroxyanisole and tocopherols.

(b) Preservatives

A preservative is a substance which is added to pharmaceutical formulations to prevent or inhibit the growth of microorganisms in the preparations. They are added to all formulations which are to be stored for long periods of time and the ingredients of which support microbial growth. The emulsions and suspensions containing water and carbohydrates as emulsifying and suspending agents respectively, must be suitably preserved because water and carbohydrates provide very good medium for the multiplication of bacterias and molds. Further, the parenteral preparations packed in multidose containers must contain a preservative to check the growth of microorganisms which may have accidentally entered the container during the withdrawal of a dose.

A preservative is unnecessary in multidose containers prepared by heating with bactericide because they already contain a lethal substance, nor they are necessary in preparations which contain medicaments having bactericidal properties.

Choice of Preservative

The preservative selected should have the following properties:

1. It should be effective against a wide range of microorganisms.
2. It should be compatible with other ingredients of the formulation.
3. It should be soluble in aqueous phase when used in emulsions.
4. It should be nontoxic.
5. It should be free from odour and taste.
6. It should preserve the prepaiations and remain stable for the shelf life of the product.

No single preservative possesses all the qualities therefore it becomes necessary to use a combination of preservatives to prevent the growth of microorganisms. The most commonly used preservatives are as follows:

1. Benzoic acid and sodium benzoate 0.1 to 0.2%.
2. Salicylic acid 0.1%.
3. Phenol 0.2 to 0.5%.
4. Chlorocresol 0.05 to 0.1%.
5. Alcohol 15 to 20%.
6. Chlorbutanol 0.5%.
7. Phenylmercuric nitrate 0.002 to 0.005%.
8. Sorbic acid and its salts 0.05 to 0.2%.
9. Benzalkonium chloride 0.004 to 0.02%.
10. Methyl paraben and propyl paraben 0.1% to 0.2%.

Colouring Agents

Colouring agents may be defined as the substances used to impart colour to foods, drugs and cosmetics to increase their organoleptic properties. In pharmaceutical preparations they may be used to increase their acceptability by the patients, to give warning, or to produce standard preparations.

Colours may be obtained from minerals, plants and animals or they can be prepared by synthesis. Colours obtained from minerals are also known as pigments. At one time they were used in cosmetics and lotions meant for external application to the skin but now a days their use is restricted and are replaced by synthetic colours. The examples of mineral colours are ferric oxide (yellow and red), carbon black, titanium dioxide and ultramarine.

Different colours obtained from plants include chlorophyll, indigo, alizarin, carotenoids and flavones. Cochineal was the only animal colour used in pharmaceutical preparations. But now a days the colours obtained from plants and animals are rarely used, they are replaced by synthetic colours.

The synthetic colours are prepared from coal tar dyes which include nitro-dyes, nitroso-dyes, azo-dyes, thiazines, rosanilines, etc. They are mainly used in textile industries. Only the permitted colours are used in food and pharmaceutical preparations. Caramel or burnt sugar, an artificial colour is used to produce brown colour in cough syrups, elixirs and other oral liquid preparations.

Amount of Colouring Agent Required

There is no hard and fast rule regarding the quantity of colouring agent used in the preparations. It depends upon the depth of colour required, the thickness of solution to be viewed and the presence of suspended powders in the preparation. An approximate quantity of colouring agent used for liquid preparations is 0.0001% to 0.001% and for powders is 0.1%.

Flavouring Agents

Flavouring agents are the substances which are used to impart pleasant smell to the preparation and to mask specific type of taste of the preparation, thus make them more palatable. Most of the flavours used in pharmaceutical preparations are obtained from natural sources but now a days they are being replaced by synthetic flavours.

There are a large number of flavouring agents which are used to impart acceptable smell to pharmaceutical preparations. Generally the preparations which are taken orally are flavoured with fruity and spicy flavours and the preparations which are applied externally are flavoured with flowery flavouring agents. The flavouring agents obtained from natural sources include pine-apple, banana, cardamom, ginger, cinnamom, peppermint and volatile oils obtained from anise, caraway, clove, dill, lemon, orange, rose, jasmine, lavender, etc. Malt extract, glycyrrihiza extract, coffee, vanilla, chocolate and tolu balsam are also used as flavouring agents. Menthol, mannitol, chloroform spirit and chloroform water are widely used as flavouring agents in liquid formulations.

Synthetic chemicals like certain alcohols, aldehydes, esters, fatty acids, ketones and lactones are used as flavouring agents. They are often preferred to natural flavouring agents because:

   (i) they are constant in composition;
  (ii) they are readily available;
 (iii) they are comparatively cheap;
 (iv) they are more stable;
  (v) their incompatibilities are more predictable.

Selection of Flavours

The problem of selection of a flavour for a particular preparation is quite complicated because flavour and taste depends on individual preferences. Moreover it depends on the qualities of the preparation which is to be flavoured. For salty preparations, cinnamon flavours are considered the best flavouring agents followed by orange syrup, cocoa syrup, wild cherry syrup and raspberry syrup. For bitter taste cocoa syrup, raspberry syrup, cherry syrup and cinnamon syrup are used. The acrid taste and sour taste can be masked by raspberry and other fruit syrups.

Oily taste of fixed oil like that of castor oil can be effectively masked with aromatic rhubarb syrup and that of cod-liver oil can be masked by oil of winter green, peppermint oil, malt extract or glycyrrihiza extract.

A blend of flavouring agents is generally used to effectively mask the odour and taste sensations. As regards the quantities of flavouring agents used in formulations, it mainly depends on the formulator. Usually 0.1 to 0.5% of volatile oil is sufficient as flavouring agent for an emulsion.

Sweetening Agents

Sweetening agents are the substances which are used in the formulations to mask the objectionable taste of the drug and make the preparation sweet in taste. Sucrose is the most widely used sweetening agent. It is obtained from sugar cane. It is quite soluble in water. It is physically and chemically stable at pH from 4.0 to 8.0. Simple syrup and liquid glucose are frequently used in liquid preparations. Sugar is also used in lozenges and in the coating of pills and tablets. The other sweetening agents include lactose, mannitol, honey, glycerin and sorbitol.

Artificial or synthetic sweetening agents like saccharin, sodium saccharin and sodium cyclamate are frequently used in the preparation of sugar free formulations. These compounds are soluble in water, alcohol and glycols. They are physically and chemically stable over a pH range of 3.0 to 8.0. A desired sweetness can be produced at much lower concentration than sucrose. Saccharin in dilute solutions is 300 times as sweet as sucrose. Saccharin sodium is used in tooth pastes and other preparations meant for oral hygiene because it is less likely to cause dental carries than carbohydrates. It is also used as a sweetening agent for many foods for diabetic persons and those who are on slimming diets.

Hospital Pharmacy

Hospital pharmacy is one of the most important departments of a hospital. Hospital pharmacy may be defined as that department of the hospital which deals with procurement, storage, compounding, dispensing, manufacturing, testing, packaging and distribution of drugs. It is also concerned with education and research in pharmaceutical services. Modern system of hospital pharmacy also provides drug information and drug monitoring service. A hospital pharmacy is controlled by professionally competent and legally qualified pharmacists.

The hospital pharmacy exerts a great deal of influence on the professional status of the hospital as well as the economics of the total operational costs of the institution because of its interrelation and interdependency of other services upon it. The department of pharmacy is typical of the majority of other departments in the hospital in that depending upon its size and services rendered it employs both professional and lay personnel, the number of which depends upon the nature of work etc.

FUNCTIONS OF HOSPITAL PHARMACY

Pharmacy is recognised as an essential hospital service in all the major hospitals. It is manned by professionally qualified pharmacists. It has been realised that only trained pharmaceutical personnel are capable of purchasing, storing, handling, pricing and dispensing of medications. It is the pharmacist who is an expert to provide all information regarding drugs to the health professions and to the public. Therefore, he acts as a link between the physician and the patient. A pharmacist is required to perform various functions in hospital pharmacy which are described below:

1. Providing specifications for the purchase of drugs, chemicals, biologicals etc.
2. Proper storing of drugs.
3. Manufacturing of pharmaceuticals which are manufactured in the hospital.
4. Dispensing and sterilizing parenteral preparations which are manufactured in the hospital.
5. Dispensing of drugs, chemicals and pharmaceutical preparations.
6. Supply of drugs and accessories to the other departments.
7. Filling and labelling of all drugs containers from which medicines are to be administered.
8. Participating in various committees of the hospital.
9. Implementing the decisions of the committees.
10. Maintaining and keeping available the approved stock of antidotes and other emergency drugs.
11. Maintaining and preparing periodic reports regarding the purchase and issue of drugs for submission to the hospital authorities.
12. Furnishing information concerning medications to the physicians, nurses or any other competent person who deals in drugs.
13. Providing cooperation in teaching and research programmes of the hospital.
14. Discarding the expired drugs and containers with worn, illegible or missing labels.

ORGANIZATION OF HOSPITAL PHARMACY

"An organization may be defined as the arrangement of persons in any field so that they act as one body and work together to fulfil the common goal". Better the organization better would be the achievement of the common objectives. Similarly loose organization would lead to unhappy and serious results. Therefore, it is the most important task of the director or the chief pharmacist to build a strong organizational structure and to fit the right person in the right place in order to achieve the goal efficiently and economically.

The organizational structure of hospital pharmacy varies with the size and complexity of the hospital. The number of lay, skilled and pharmacy personnel cannot be determined unless some thought is given to the nature of services to be rendered to the various departments i.e. is the department to serve in-patients and/or out-patients and how many per day? Is there to be a manufacturing section of pharmacy and what type of formulations are to be manufactured?

A director or chief pharmacist should be the incharge of hospital pharmacy who should be professionally competent and legally qualified. He should be minimum graduate in pharmacy from a recognised college of pharmacy. The director should be assisted by additional qualified pharmacists and skilled personnel as needed according to the nature of work. Trained pharmacy assistants should not be assigned the duties which are required to be performed only by the registered pharmacists. Clerical staff should be provided as needed to assist in the smooth working of the pharmacy.

In any hospital all the individuals and organizations are coordinated primarily to provide the best medical facilities to the hospital patients.

Location

The pharmacy should be centrally located in the hospital so that patients and staff can easily approach it. In multistoreyed building of a hospital, the pharmacy should be preferably located on the ground floor specially the dispensing unit. The out-patient department should give positive impression to the patients.

Planning

Before starting any hospital pharmacy it is very important to plan the things. Without sound planning it is very difficult to achieve the desired aims. Therefore, a sound thinking must be given that what is to be done, when and where it is to be done and how it is to be done according to the funds available? What type of products are to be formulated, type of building and equipment required? The number of pharmacists, skilled and lay personnel required, their salary etc.? Provisions for the supply of good quality of raw materials and finished products and facilities for the testing of these materials.

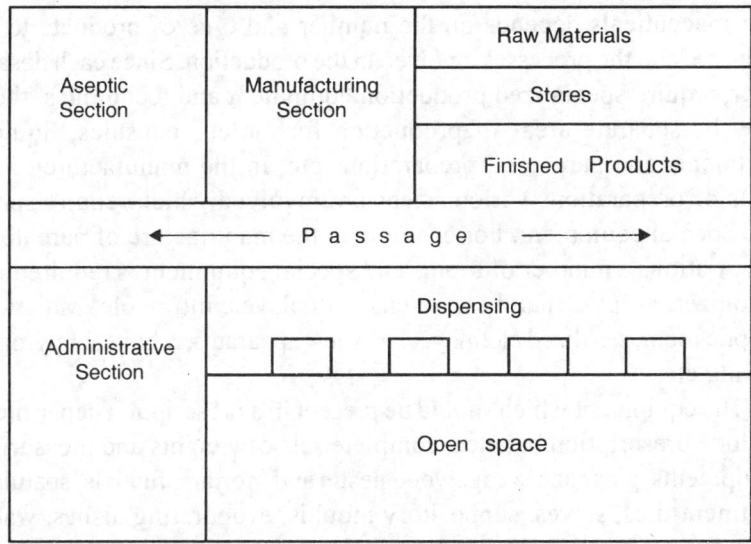

Fig. 12.1. Typical layout of hospital pharmacy.

Staff of Hospital Pharmacy

It depends on the number of beds in the hospital, services rendered to the out-patients and indoor patients whether it is involved in manufacturing of drugs and formations.

The staff of hospital pharmacy comprises of registered pharmacists, skilled persons, lay persons and clerical staff. All the staff members must know their duties and place of work. They should discharge their duties and responsibilities in the best way because all of them are engaged in the health care of the patient is one way or the other. All the employees must have good relations with both intra- and interdepartmental employees.

A well-qualified pharmacist must have a thorough knowledge regarding drugs and their actions. He should be able to undertake manufacturing of pharmaceutical products. At the same time he should have knowledge regarding the analytical procedures of drugs. He should be able to conduct teaching and research work. He should have good command and able to administer and manage a hospital pharmacy.

Space and Equipment

The space and equipment required for the manufacture of

pharmaceuticals depends on the number and type of products to be prepared and the processes involved in the production. Since each dosage form require specialized production equipment and techniques, there may be separate areas of production for tablets, capsules, liquids, ointments and parenteral preparations etc. In the manufacture of all sorts of preparations various steps are involved which require space and special equipment. For example in the manufacture of parenteral preparations a number of rooms and special equipment is required i.e. deionizer, aseptic chambers, ovens, autoclaves, ultraviolet radiation, aseptic room, sterilized clothing, clarity test apparatus, rabbits for pyrogen testing etc.

The equipment which should be present in a prescription department include prescription balance, complete sets of weights and measuring equipments, glass and wedgewood pestle and mortars, funnels, spatulas, ointment tiles, sieves, suppository moulds, evaporating dishes, water bath, thermometers, glass rods etc.

In general the drugs must be stored under proper conditions so as to preserve their stability and therapeutic effectiveness. For storing the drug in a cool place, a refrigerator should be provided in the pharmacy. The latest literature of pharmaceutical education should be provided so that pharmacists and nursing staff may have up to date knowledge of drugs.

PHARMACEUTICAL SERVICES IN OUT-PATIENT DEPARTMENT

In short form the out-patient department is known as OPD. The patient with minor and common illness go to the OPD for consultation to the physician. After examining the patient if the physician feels that there is no need of admitting the patient to the hospital ward, he prescribes the medicines. The patient is required to get the prescribed medicines from the hospital pharmacy and take home these medicines. If the need arises he can again go to OPD and consult the physician.

The prescription written by the physician is brought to the pharmacist for compounding and dispensing. After careful examination of the prescription, the pharmacist carry out the compounding. The compounded medicaments are filled into suitable containers which are labelled properly. The pharmacist also calculates the price of the filled prescription. After receiving the payment the filled prescription is handed over to the patient. The prescriptions are then filled into regular prescription file or the narcotic prescription file as the case may be. The pharmacist also prepares the statistics and reports regarding the filled prescriptions.

Location of Out-patient Dispensing Area

There is no set rule regarding the location of out-patient dispensing area, preferably it should be located on the ground floor of the building and near to the entrance of the building for easy access by the patients. It should be close to the central registration and out-patient departments so that the patients do not find any difficulty in its location.

The out-patient dispensing area should be provided with proper seating arrangement so that if long time is needed for filling the prescription, the patient can wait till the prescription is filled.

Receipt system

Drugs in a hospital pharmacy may be obtained from one or more than one sources as describes below:

1. Direct from the manufacturer.
2. Direct from the wholeseller.

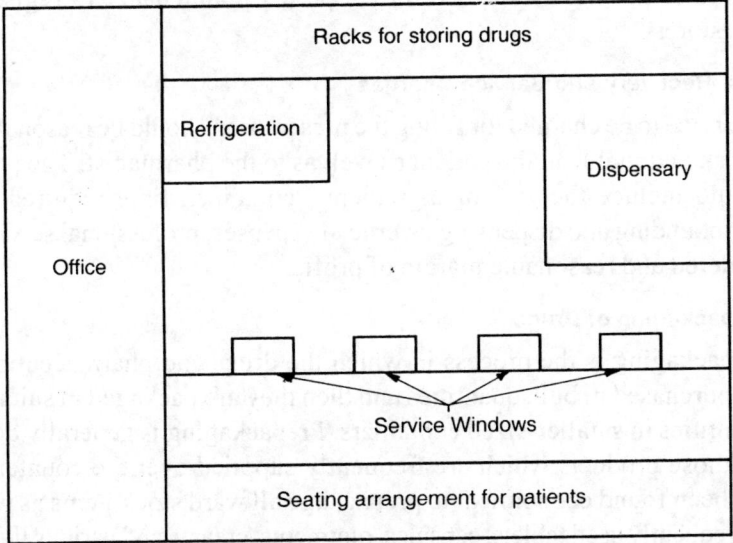

Fig. 12.2. Typical layout of an OPD.

3. By inviting the tenders.
4. From local retail pharmacy.
5. Through agents.
6. Through a hospital purchase centre or corporation.
7. From local manufacturing unit of the hospital.

For the purchase or receipt of medicaments the requirement is noted in the prescribed forms in which the complete data regarding description, specification, packaging, price and quantity needed is given. Three copies of requirement are prepared out of which one copy is sent to the supplier, second to the accounts office and the third is retained by the pharmacy. After receiving the supplies each and every item is entered separately in the receipt register which is properly maintained and countersigned by the superior officer. The maintenance of register gives ready reference for source of supply, cost of drug, quantity in hand etc.

Issue system

No medicament should be issued without the proper prescription written by a competent medical officer. After the issue has been made the quantities supplied must be recorded in the issue register. A proper account must be maintained regarding the quantity received and the quantity issued. The difference gives the balance quantity in hand which should be physically verified for the proper maintenance of registers and stores.

Cost Recovery and Service Charges

The price to be charged for filling the prescription should be reasonable, fair and equitable to the patient as well as to the pharmacist. The price should include the cost of ingredients, container, time required for compounding and dispensing, overhead expenses, professional services rendered and reasonable margin of profit.

Prepackaging of Drugs

Prepackaging is the process in which the drugs and pharmaceuticals are purchased in bulk quantities and then they are packaged in suitable quantities in smaller-sized containers. Prepackaging is generally done for those products which are frequently supplied over the counter. It has been found economical to prepackage all ward stock items as well as frequently used tablets, capsules, ointments, creams and various liquid preparations. Tablets and capsules can be prepackaged in small containers of 12's, 24's, 48's, 100's etc. Similarly liquids can also be prepackaged in small containers. Prepacking can be done for both out-patients as well as in-patients. It increases the efficiency of the pharmacy department. Each prepackaged container must be properly labelled.

Factors Determining Pack Size

There are no hard and fast rules for determining the pack size of a product. It depends on the local situation and the demand of a particular product. Some of the factors which must be considered in determining the pack size are:

1. Demand for the product i.e. whether the product is required daily, occasionally or seasonally. For example analgesics, antacids, anthelmintics, laxatives, antibiotics and tonics are required throughout the year whereas antimalarials are required seasonally.
2. How many units are to be packaged and total number of packages to be prepared?
3. What type of containers should be used so as to maintain therapeutic properties of the preparation?
4. Can the product be packaged by hand or by machine?
5. Is there any special label required?
6. What are the conditions required for the stability of the product?
7. Will the pre-packing be economical or not and what will be the cost of prepackaged product?

On small scale, prepackaging can be done by hand but on large scale it can be done mechanically. Hospitals which require large scale prepackaging operations have installed separate units for this purpose. Prepackaging operation must be carried out by a pharmacist with the assistance of a helper.

PHARMACEUTICAL SERVICES IN IN-PATIENT DEPARTMENT

The drug distribution to the in-patient departments can be carried out from the out-patient dispensing area. The staff handling the distribution of drugs to out-patients can carry-out the distribution of drugs to in-patient departments. If work load is too much additional personnel may be employed. This system will be economical as extra expenditure on building and staff will be saved. Moreover this system has additional advantage that the director or chief pharmacist can exert a great degree of control and supervision of the activities of the department.

Separate drug distribution area for in-patient departments can be set up on the ground floor or first floor of the building but it should be near the in-patient departments and centrally located so that the staff can easily reach there. The in-patient dispensing should be carried out by a pharmacist helped by skilled and lay personnel.

Drug Distribution Systems

In an in-patient department, the physician prescribes, the pharmacist dispenses and usually the nurses administer the drug. To carry out this process a number of procedures, personnel, departments, equipments etc. are involved. So there are a number of systems by which drugs can be distributed to the in-patient departments but all the systems are deficit in one way or the other. Now a days there are four systems by which the drugs are distributed for in-patients which are described below:

1. Individual prescription order system.
2. Complete floor stock system.
3. A combination of number 1 and 2.
4. Unit dose dispensing.

The first three methods are considered poor drug control methods as compared to No. 4.

1. Individual prescription order system

This system is generally used in small and/or private hospitals because of its revenue production and reduced manpower requirements. This system has the advantages that (i) all the medication orders are directly reviewed by the pharmacist so there are less medication errors (ii) it provides closer liaison among pharmacist, physician, nurse and the patient in the medication matters, (iii) it provides closer control of inventory.

This system has certain disadvantages that (i) there may be possible delay in obtaining the required medications for administration to the patient, (ii) increase in the cost to the patient.

2. Complete floor stock system

According to this system the drugs are stored at the nursing stations and are administered by a nurse according to the chart order of the physician. Only the commonly used drugs in considerable quantities are stocked on the floor (complete floor stock) or on the ward (ward stock).

Rarely used or costly drugs are not included in the floor stock but are dispensed when the order is received for the individual patients. Mainly this system is used in hospitals where the charges are not made to patients.

Since these drugs are used in large quantities they are prepackaged in standard containers. Nursing staff from each floor or ward sends their written demand of drugs and other items according to the list provided to each floor and ward, daily, to the hospital pharmacy herself or through a messenger who will collect the medications from the pharmacist.

This system has the advantages (i) the drugs are readily available for administration, (ii) minimum return of drugs, (iii) reduced in-patient prescription orders, (iv) reduction in the number of pharmacy personnel required.

The disadvantages of this system include:

 (i) Increase in chances of medication errors due to lack of review by pharmacists.
 (ii) Greater opportunity for misappropriation of medication resulting in financial loss.
(iii) Increase in drug inventory.
(iv) Increased chances of drug deterioration due to lack of proper storage facilities.
 (v) Increased danger of drug hazards due to unnoticed drug deterioration.
(vi) Increased work load on nurses due to medication activities.

3. Combination of systems

This system is used in those hospitals where the patients pay for their hospitalization and the hospitals use the individual prescription order system as their primary means of dispensing but have several drugs in the floor stock. This system is most commonly used for drug distribution in hospitals.

4. Unit dose dispensing

In unit dose dispensing the multiples of single dose administration of medication are prepared by the pharmacist which are ready for administration to a particular patient, by the prescribed route and at the prescribed time rather than supplying containers of drugs to nursing units where the nurse is required to prepare the drug for administration. A single unit package is one which contains one complete pharmaceutical dosage form, e.g. one tablet, one capsule or 10 ml of oral liquid. Liquids are premeasured, powders accurately weighed and diluted, parenteral preparations are suitably diluted and accurately measured into sterile syringes ready for administration. Each single unit package is labelled for each patient with appropriate directions.

Advantages of Unit Dose Dispensing
1. The medications are readily available to the patients and they are charged for only those doses which are administered to them.
2. Medication errors are decreased because of direct check by the pharmacist.
3. Drugs are easily identifiable for individual patients.
4. Contamination due to handling is eliminated.
5. Since all doses are prepared by the hospital pharmacy, it eliminates the "pouring" time of nurses thus allowing them more time for direct patient care.
6. It eliminates wastage of drugs.

Disadvantages of Unit Dose Dispensing
1. It requires more space since the packaging material increases the bulk of the dosage form.
2. It requires increased number of skilled and lay personnel in the pharmacy.
3. The cost of medication is increased to the patient due to increased handling charges.

Unit dose dispensing can be carried out through the use of strip packaging, blister packaging, vials and disposable syringes. Tablets or capsules can be pre-packaged in strips or blisters each containing 5 to 10 tablets or capsules. Vials may be filled with 15, 30 or 60 ml liquid medication. Injectables may be filled in disposable glass syringes which are commercially available in 0.5, 1.0, 2.0, 5.0 and 10 ml sizes.

Maintenance of records of issue and use of narcotics and dangerous drugs

The narcotics and dangerous drugs must be issued on narcotic prescription order form which must bear the date, full name, age, address and registration number of the patient. It must be signed by the authorised practitioner. His full address and registration number must be there on the prescription. The prescription order must bear the name, strength and quantity of drug to be supplied as well as the directions for its use. The narcotic prescriptions must be filled on the same date when they are written. A proper record regarding the receipt and issue of narcotics must be maintained. A separate register must be used for this purpose.

Ward stock medicines

Ward stock medicines consist of a predetermined list of medications which are available in the ward. The list of such medicines which are used on a ward is prepared by Pharmacy and Therapeutics Committee. Once the list of medications has been determined, it becomes the responsibility of the hospital pharmacist to make the drugs available on the ward. The nursing matron should maintain the stock according to the need of the ward. Whenever need arises for more medicines she should get them from hospital pharmacy by sending written demand. A proper record must be maintained by the nurse for the receipt and issue of medications.

Emergency drugs

Emergency drugs should be made available on the ward to meet any emergency needs. The Pharmacy and Therapeutics Committee should determine the list of emergency drugs. Once the list of emergency drugs is determined it becomes the joint responsibility of the pharmacist and the nurse to have the box containing these drugs ready for use at all times. The box must be checked periodically to ensure that all the recommended drugs are available in sufficient quantities to meet any emergency.

Routine inspection of drug stocks in wards

It is the responsibility of hospital pharmacist to inspect various wards of the hospital and see that:
1. Drugs are stored properly and their stability maintained.
2. Drugs are available according to the needs of the patients and in sufficient quantities.
3. Poisons are stored separately under lock.
4. Proper records are maintained regarding the receipt and issue of medications.

5. Balance quantities of drugs shown in the register are physically present in the stock.
6. Emergency boxes contain the specified drugs in sufficient amounts.
7. The drugs not consumed are returned to the pharmacy.

MEDICAL STORES

Medical stores are the places where the drugs are stored for distribution to the hospital wards and other user departments. They are handled by competent and legally qualified pharmacists assisted by trained personnel.

Objectives

Medical stores has the following objectives:

1. To stock all drugs and accessories required in the hospital.
2. To procure drugs from the different sources.
3. To supply drugs to the consuming departments.
4. To store drugs required in research work.
5. To preserve certain categories of drugs.
6. To maintain records of receipt and issue of drugs.
7. To carry out all the operations regarding drugs economically to save revenue.

Layout and facilities

The medical stores should be centrally located in a spacious and well ventilated building. The rooms should be fitted with shelves and drawers made up of wood or steel. Space should be provided for a refrigerator. A trolley should be provided for transporting heavy articles.

In order that the pharmacist may properly supervise the storage of drugs, they should be stored in an area directly under his control. In this way he will be able to arrange the stocks according to his knowledge as well as according to the prescribing trends of the staff. All procurements made by pharmacy should directly reach the pharmacy area. If the merchandise are received by the hospital post office or central store room, it should be immediately forwarded to the medical stores in the unopened state. After receiving the merchandise in the stores, the pharmacy personnel are required to check the materials physically with the receiving slip and with the copy of the purchase order. The materials received must be entered in the receipt register.

All the medicines and accessories must be put on the shelves. The fast moving items must be kept handy near the counter. The slow moving drugs or the drugs which are not used frequently may be kept on the upper shelves. The bulky items should be kept on the bottom shelves. The accessories and other equipments like surgical instruments, rubber goods and sutures should be stored separately on racks specially reserved for the purpose.

There is no specific rule by which the drugs should be arranged in a store. It depends on the individual who is to handle the store. The arrangement should meet his and the institutional requirements. Generally the drugs may be arranged according to their categories or according to the companies who has supplied the drugs. But they must be arranged alphabetically on the shelves.

Procedure for procurement of drugs and supplies from the medical stores depot

The drugs and supplies are procured from the Medical Store Depot (MSD) by the hospitals, institutions and stores by sending the requisition to the depot manager of the Medical Store Depot. Each and every item have been allotted VMS No. (Vocabulary of Medical Stores No.) which must be given while filling the indent form. Complete specifications and unit pack size must also be mentioned. If specifications regarding drug items are not mentioned then the pharmacopoeial standard drugs are supplied to the indentors.

Three copies of the indent form are sent to Medical Store Depot and fourth copy is retained by the indentor. After verifying the stock position of the stores, two copies of the indent are sent back to the indentor mentioning the price of the drugs etc.

After the amount is deposited in advance by the indentor with the Medical Store Depot, the drugs are supplied to the indentor. On receipt of the drugs/supplies, the materials are verified by the indentor regarding the quality and quantity. Then they are entered into the receipt register and the drugs/supplies stored in the stores.

Procurement of drugs from manufacturers/distributors

Drugs can be procured directly from the manufacturers are on the list of approved suppliers. Three copies of the requisition are prepared. One copy is retained by the indentor and two are sent to the manufacturer. Complete specifications, unit and price must be mentioned according to the lists of drugs/materials supplied, from time to time, by the manufacturers.

After receiving the orders, the supplies are made to the indenting department, institution or hospital by the manufacturer on the receipt of the drugs/supplies the materials are verified by the indentor regarding the quality and quantity of drugs supplied. If found correct, a certificate is given and bills passed for payment. The drugs supplies are entered in the receipt register and stores in stores.

Some manufacturers do not supply the drugs directly to the user departments but they appoint their own distributors who supplies the drugs to indenting departments. The procedure regarding the procurement of drugs/supplies is the same as described in the procedure for procurement of drugs from manufacturers.

Procurement of drugs from local market

The drugs and materials which are urgently required or are required in small quantities can be purchases from the local market by an authorised person against cash payment or credit.

Procedure and limits for emergency purchases

Emergency purchases of drugs are made when they are not in stores and they are urgently required. The prescriber must mention that these are life saving drugs and are urgently required for a particular patient and for a particular disease. Only then the drugs are purchased from the local market against cash payment or credit. A pharmacist must be authorised to do the emergency purchases as and when required.

LICENSING PROCEDURE FOR PROCURING AND STOCKING OF ALCOHOL AND NARCOTICS

A licence is necessary for the procurement and stocking of alcohol and other narcotics. The applicant will have to apply to the excise commissioner of the concerned state along with the prescribed fee. The application should include the following information:

1. Name and address of the applicant and the place at which the alcohol is to be stocked.
2. The purpose for which the alcohol is required.
3. The quantity of alcohol required.

If after making the enquiries the licensing authority is satisfied, may issue the licence for the procurement of alcohol. He may direct a particular distillery or spirit warehouse from where alcohol can be obtained. After depositing the amount and excise duty the excise officer-incharge of the distillery shall issue the spirit in a sealed container along with a permit covering the issue. The spirit so obtained should be immediately transferred to the spirit store and necessary entries made in the register maintained for the purpose. A proper record for the receipt and issue of alcohol must be maintained and the stock register must be verified by the concerned excise inspector.

Sampling for quality control

The excise officer in whose jurisdiction the premises is located, without previous notice to the manufacturer may inspect the premises and take samples at random of not less than 10% and not more than 15% of the total number of batches manufactured during the month. All such samples should be taken by the excise officer himself in the presence of the manufacturer. All samples should be taken in duplicate and labels of all containers signed by the officer. The samples so collected must be seated immediately by fixing a seal of the officer concerned. If the manufacturer so desires he may also put his signatures on the labels of the containers and fix his own seal along with the seal of the officer on the containers. The sealed samples are then sent to the chemical examiner for analysis.

Disposal of slow moving drugs

Slow moving drugs may be regarded as those drugs which are rarely prescribed, therefore, occasionally dispensed over the counter. Slow moving drugs should not be stocked in the store. Orders for such drugs should be carefully placed. They should be procured only when the stock already in hand is about to finish. If large quantities of slow moving drugs have piled up in the store, they can be disposed off as follows:

1. They can be donated to charitable hospitals.
2. They can be replaced with the fresh stock from the manufacturers.
3. They can be sold to local dealers.
4. They can be distributed free of cost to the needy persons.
5. If there is no other way out for their disposal they may be destroyed with the permission of the authorities and written off from the stock register.

Dead stock

These are the drugs which become unfit for human consumption due to one reason or the other. They may have been deteriorated due to atmospheric conditions, improper storage conditions, some formulation defects or they may have expired the shelf life of the drug. Such drugs must be stored in separate cupboards labelled "Expired Drugs". Such drugs must be destroyed with the permission of the authorities and written off from the stock register. The drugs which can be reprocessed may be sent to the manufacturers for reprocessing.

Reference Books

1. Remington's Pharmaceutical Sciences, Mack Publishing Company, Pennsylvania.
2. Dispensing of Medication, Formerly Husa's Pharmaceutical Dispensing, Mack Publishing Co., Easton, Pennsylvania.
3. The Theory and Practice of Industrial Pharmacy, Lea and Febiger, Philadelphia.
4. Cooper and Gunn's Dispensing for Pharmaceutical Students, CBS Publishers & Distributors, New Delhi, India.
5. Clinical Pharmacy : A Text For Dispensing Pharmacy, Jenkins, Sperandio and Latiolais, McGraw-Hill Book Company, London.
6. Mithal : Text Book of Pharmaceutical Formulations, Birla Institute of Technology and Science, Pilani.
7. Schroff : Professional Pharmacy, Part V, Vol. I, National Book Centre, Dr. Sundari Mohan Avenue, Calcutta - 14.
8. Schroff : Professional Pharmacy, Part V, Vol. II, Five Stars Enterprises, Dr. Sundari Mohan Avenue, Calcutta - 14.
9. The Pharmacopoeia of India.
10. National Formulary of India.
11. The British Pharmacopoeia.
12. British Pharmaceutical Codex.

13. The Pharmacopoeia of United States.
14. Extra Pharmacopoeia Martindale.
15. The Pharmacopoeia of U.S.S.R.
16. Ansel: Introduction to Pharmaceutical Dosage Forms.
17. William E. Hassan: Hospital Pharmacy, Lea and Febiger, Philadelphia.
18. Australian Pharmaceutical Formulary and Handbook, Pharmaceutical Society of Australia.

Index